I'm Not That Person Anymore

A Nurse's Journey Living With Metastatic Breast Cancer

by
Elizabeth Wertz Evans, PhD, RN, MPM, CPHQ, CPHIMS, FHIMSS, FACMPE,
and Anne Katz, PhD, RN, FAAN

Hygeia Media
An imprint of the Oncology Nursing Society
Pittsburgh, Pennsylvania

ONS Publications Department

Publisher and Director of Publications: William A. Tony, BA, CQIA
Managing Editor: Lisa M. George, BA
Assistant Managing Editor: Amy Nicoletti, BA, JD
Acquisitions Editor: John Zaphyr, BA, MEd
Copy Editors: Vanessa Kattouf, BA, Andrew Petyak, BA
Graphic Designer: Dany Sjoen
Editorial Assistant: Judy Holmes

Library of Congress Cataloging-in-Publication Data

Names: Wertz Evans, Elizabeth, author. | Katz, Anne (Anne Jennifer), 1958-
author.
Title: I'm not that person anymore : a nurse's journey living with metastatic
breast cancer / by Elizabeth Wertz Evans, PhD, RN, MPM, CPHQ, CPHIMS,
FHIMSS, FACMPE, and Anne Katz, PhD, RN, FAAN.
Description: Pittsburgh, Pennsylvania : Hygeia Media, an imprint of the
Oncology Nursing Society, 2016. | Includes bibliographical references.
Identifiers: LCCN 2016016350 (print) | LCCN 2016025701 (ebook) | ISBN
9781935864851 | ISBN 9781935864868 (pdf) | ISBN 9781935864875 (epub)
Subjects: LCSH: Wertz Evans, Elizabeth--Health. |
Breast--Cancer--Patients--United States--Biography. |
Metastasis--Patients--United States--Biography. | Nurses--Biography.
Classification: LCC RC280.B8 W417 2016 (print) | LCC RC280.B8 (ebook) | DDC
362.19699/4490092 [B] --dc23
LC record available at https://lccn.loc.gov/2016016350

Publisher's Note

Printed in the United States of America

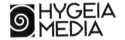

An imprint of the Oncology Nursing Society

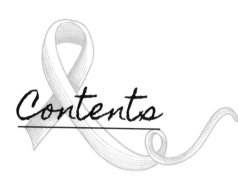

Contents

Acknowledgments

I am blessed to have such wonderful, supportive family and friends.

Sandy has been my best friend since we graduated high school together in 1974. We have been breast cancer warriors/sisters since 2009. She had her first breast cancer diagnosis more than 10 years ago and was treated with surgery, chemotherapy, and radiation. It still amazes me that both of us are living in this world. She lives in Clearfield, Pennsylvania, and has three grown daughters and two granddaughters. Clearfield is about three hours from Pittsburgh. Whenever we'd go to Penn State University to watch Ashley W. cheer, we would stop to visit her or stay with her for the weekend. In fact, we go to a breast cancer awareness girls' basketball game at Penn State together every year. We each get a pink survivor T-shirt. The basketball team members wear pink uniforms, and the cheerleaders have bright pink bows in their hair. All of the survivors then go down to the court at halftime and are honored. The first time I went, Ashley W. was a cheerleader. I hugged her as I came off the floor. We both tried so hard not to cry.

My friend Sharon and I met in 1978 in nursing school. We did lots of projects together and became best friends after graduating in May 1980. She has two boys, a girl, and multiple grandchildren. Her children call me "Aunt Liz," and my kids call her "Aunt Sharon." I always feel like a member of her family and vice versa. We joke around about someday being in a nursing home together.

Several of my friends and I go out to dinner every so often, which really helps my mental health. We all met almost 20 years ago as

Bunco Babes. We used to actually play the game at one another's houses. Now, because everyone is so busy, we get together, go to dinner, and talk about life. Several of the girls are starting to become grandparents, so it gives us a chance to catch up with what is going on in their lives. A few of them were helpful in "escorting" me to my chemotherapy treatments, as I could not drive with the narcotics I was taking. They all are so dear to me.

Thank you also to Ginny Pribanic from MedResponse (www .medresponse.com), who provided some funding for the book's promotional video. It turned out great! Thanks also to Mary Anne Van Develde, who did most of the video filming.

Thanks to Andrew Petyak, John Zaphyr, Lisa George, Dany Sjoen, and Bill Tony from the ONS Publications Department for their undying support and work on the project. I am so grateful.

—*Liz Wertz Evans*

While Liz and I collaborated on this book, there were others who also made it happen. John Zaphyr, the acquisitions editor for the Oncology Nursing Society, has worked with me on many books over the past 10 years. His support, encouragement, and dedication to Liz's story deserve special recognition and my personal gratitude.

—*Anne Katz*

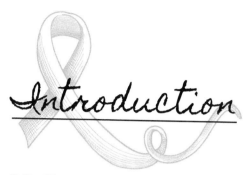

Introduction

My Story

I was at the top of my game.

I was an executive director leading my staff at the Oncology Nursing Society (ONS). I was putting the finishing touches on my PhD, traveling around the country as a representative of ONS, and serving as a key member on several committees. Basically, I was taking the world by storm.

Then, this devil called metastatic cancer showed up and immediately stopped me in my tracks.

So, how did I get here? Why did I write this book?

In the pages to follow, you will read about this journey. I will share with you my personal journal entries from my first diagnosis of breast cancer to its recurrence nearly five years later. The entries are personal, they are raw and unvarnished, and they represent me. To help guide you, I have recruited Anne Katz, PhD, RN, FAAN, an author of several best-selling books on cancer, to make sense of everything. She will explain the evidence and science behind my experiences and provide insight into what it is like for a woman who is a nurse *LIVING* with metastatic cancer.

So, again, why exactly did I write this book? Was it to become famous? No. To quit my full-time job and live off of the royalties? Ha! I don't think so!

My hope is that this book helps other patients fighting metastatic breast cancer, as well as the nurses who take care of them.

Family First

As you will see in this introduction, family is very important to me. My nuclear family is first on the list, followed by aunts, uncles, and cousins. I don't have many of the latter, so it's not too hard to keep track of everyone.

I grew up in a northern suburb of Pittsburgh with my parents Bill and Helen, my sister Patty, and my brother Charlie, the baby of the family. We had a wonderful childhood. Sure, we fought as kids, just as siblings often do, but as we grew up, matured, and experienced the good and bad things about life, we always supported one another.

Patty and I are very close. She has been a true advocate for me and comes to almost every one of my doctor's appointments. In fact, she usually shows up before I do!

She has plans to remarry and asked me to be her matron of honor. (She has been mine several times!) Of course, I accepted! I pray that I still will be alive and active by the time the wedding rolls around.

At 23 years old, I moved out of the house and married my high school sweetheart on June 30, 1979. The marriage lasted about two years. My mother was right—I would not be able to change things just because we were married.

I was in nursing school when I met my second husband, Patrick L. Wertz. He also was a nursing student but in the class below me. I graduated in 1980 and he in 1981. At school, our relationship blossomed. We especially loved working together in the cardiovascular intensive care unit (CVICU).

A few years after graduating, we got married on May 7, 1983. We had three children: Patrick, Amanda, and Ashley.

Pat was very involved in our children's lives and was a terrific dad. He coached baseball for Patrick's teams and softball for Ashley's teams. We did a lot of things together, even with Amanda's disability. We took her everywhere!

My son, Patrick Fitzgerald Wertz, was my first-born child on May 19, 1984. He was a great kid and very easy to raise. He graduated from Duquesne University in 2015 with a bachelor's degree in psychology and sociology. He now is working full time at Duquesne in their Information Systems Management Department. He's also considering law school.

My first daughter, Amanda Elizabeth Wertz, was born on June 11, 1987. Amanda was a special child. She provided us with many challenges and joys and taught us so many things about people with disabilities. Sadly, her life was cut short. More on this tragedy shortly.

My second daughter, Ashley Marie Wertz, was born on September 2, 1992. I am so proud of the woman she has become. She's had to deal with several challenging events in her life. At a young age, she was involved in a car crash, suffering multiple injuries as well as the loss of her father. Through an intensive year of physical rehabilitation, she regained her ability to walk and something else she had lost—her spot cheering on the sidelines.

Ashley loves cheering. She loves it so much that she stuck with it through college. When she wasn't cheering on the Penn State Nittany Lions football team from the sidelines at Beaver Stadium, she was working toward a bachelor's degree in biobehavioral health. She graduated in 2015.

Today, she is following in my footsteps; she currently is working as a certified nursing assistant until she gets into a nursing school to become an RN.

My Amanda

Ten weeks into Amanda's life, she began to have seizures and was admitted to the ICU for three weeks. The pediatricians brought in a neurologist to help diagnose her. She was found to have infantile spasms, a type of epilepsy.

She lost any milestones she had gained to that point.

The doctors put her in a phenobarbital coma until they could finalize her medications. They put her on steroids, which gave her a ferocious appetite and big chubby cheeks. When we finally took her home, we put a schedule on the refrigerator to remember what meds to give her and when. We were giving her adrenocorticotropic hormone injections in her legs twice per day in addition to other meds that treated the side effects of the steroid. The seizures finally stopped, at least temporarily. I started working from home two days per week to take care of Amanda. When I'd go into the office, my nursing friends would attend to her.

Her diagnosis of infantile spasms (the most serious form of epilepsy) occurred at 10 weeks of age. She went on to have a history of refractory seizures (meaning they could not be controlled) as well as Lennox-Gastaut syndrome. She had only one year of her life in which she did NOT have seizures. Falling from the seizures resulted in numerous injuries and frequent trips to the emergency department (ED) for stitches. It was routine to see her have 10–20 minute clusters of seizures four or five times per day. Despite her disability, however, she still was a valued member of our family.

We did our best to turn her disability into a way to educate. I did multiple lectures for emergency medical technicians, paramedics, nurses, and physicians on how to care for children with special healthcare needs. Many times, my husband would walk Amanda into a lecture hall so attendees could see that she was just a regular child. I also got involved with the Epilepsy Foundation of Western/Central Pennsylvania (EFWCP) (www.efwp.org). Through EFWCP, I was on a Listserv with other parents to share ideas and offer general support.

At times, it was very difficult to communicate with Amanda, as she could not tell us what was wrong. She would laugh when she was happy and grunt or cry when she was upset. As a young child, she would sign with her hands, which made us feel like we had a secret language. Even the kids at her daycare center learned the signs. It was fun to see them all adjust to this different child sitting at the same table with them. It was inclusion at its finest! Unfortunately, that skill disappeared as the seizures increased.

As time passed, the seizures and meds she needed took a significant toll on her development. At 14 years old, Amanda could not speak and had an estimated developmental level of 12–24 months. She wore a diaper and was fed through a special tube in her stomach.

Amanda had experimental meds, was on the ketogenic diet for about two years, and had a corpus callosotomy, where they cut her brain in half to stop the seizures. The year that she died, she had a vagus nerve stimulator implanted to help decrease the seizures. Because of these seizures and her complex medical problems, it was a challenge for us every day. Yet, seeing her seizing and caring for her just became part of our daily routine. However, I will admit that taking care of her and protecting her from harm was hard work.

Amanda also developed scoliosis (curvature of the spine) because of her low muscle tone. For many years, we took her to see a pediatric orthopedic surgeon. He was (and still is) a wonderful man. On November 8, 2001, she had her back fused and received bone grafting at a tertiary, nonpediatric hospital. The operation took a long time but was completely uneventful. She had no complications and got to the pediatric ICU around 5 pm that same day. She did well through the evening and overnight. At 6 am on November 9 (approximately 22 hours postoperation), Amanda experienced cardiac arrest (no breathing and then her heart stopped) while being suctioned through her nose. Nasal suctioning may cause cardiac dysrhythmia, including a severely slowed heart rate, or bradycardia. She was resuscitated but had no brain function. Amanda was officially pronounced dead at 1:52 pm. We made the decision to donate all viable organs. The organ harvest was completed around 7 am on November 10.

Well, we were angry for several years. We could not believe our child could be treated so incompetently and did not want the same thing happening to another family. If someone would have just said, "I'm so sorry for what happened to Amanda," we could have slept better at night. We still had complete faith in the surgeon and did not blame him at all because he did everything he could. It was the postoperative care that was horrendous and caused her death.

We decided to turn our grief into something more positive. We created various memorials and projects in Amanda's memory. I developed presentations, articles, and book chapters on the death of a child and how medical professionals could treat families in a more positive way. We tried to focus on the lives of the people that were helped by the donations of her organs and tissues.

In June 2009, we met Dayna, who was the recipient of Amanda's liver. We became close with Dayna and her family. In the spring of 2014, Dayna's new liver started to fail. I didn't know anything about it because I was in and out of the hospital for chemotherapy. On August 9, 2014, Dayna died at 25 years old due to liver failure. It was very sad. She lived near Detroit, Michigan, and my kids went there for the funeral. I was too sick to travel. My son Patrick even served as a pallbearer. I keep her picture on my "Amanda shrine" to remind us of the extra 13 years Dayna had because of Amanda.

For more information on Amanda, please check out www.panda -llc.com. There is a link to her section on the upper-right corner of the website.

Our Tragedy

On December 10, 2003, we attended a memorial service at the Highmark Caring Place (www.highmarkcaringplace.com) to remember Amanda. We were quite tearful and appreciated the love in that room. Pat and I drove separate cars, as he worked at Highmark and I was coming from our house with Ashley.

After the service, Ashley wanted to ride back home with her dad, so I told them I would see them there. I was driving behind their car but lost sight of them as we moved along the interstate. It was raining that night, and Pat was driving fast. His car hydroplaned and careened 40 feet down an embankment. I drove past the crash site and didn't know anything had happened, as his car was below a bridge.

I went home and made something for dinner. I couldn't understand why they were so late, as they had a head start on me. That's when the hospital called.

Pat was killed in the crash at the young age of 42, despite having a seat belt on. They landed with the wheels down, and Pat's head hit the cement barrier. He died immediately. He had been at the top of his game as a vice president at Highmark (Pittsburgh's Blue Cross Blue Shield organization). Suddenly, he was gone from our lives.

When I arrived in the ED at the Children's Hospital of Pittsburgh (CHP) of UPMC, Ashley was completely immobilized and conscious. She was in the front passenger seat when they crashed, which I had told her and Pat was inappropriate because she was so small. The first thing she said to me was, "I moved the seat back so the air bag would not hit me." If she had not had her seat belt on, she would have been thrown out the windshield or side window. She had bilateral femur fractures, pelvic fractures, a concussion, and a broken left hand.

Ashley was nine years old when her sister died. Now, at 11 years old, she had suffered the loss of her father. She told me she kept saying, "Please don't die, Daddy." His body was slouched in his seat from the force of the collision. His blood was all over her hair. She saw his blood-soaked face and heard his last gurgling, agonal words.

I didn't tell her about his death for about three days. She just had surgery and was in such physical pain that she was groggy most of the time from the pain meds. Patrick and his girlfriend, Stephanie, were in the room when I finally told her.

Ashley said I had lied to her about her father. I said that I had not and explained that she asked if he was OK. I said that he was, believing that Pat was in heaven with Amanda. It was so very difficult, as she was so close with her dad.

On December 11, I took a leave of absence from my full-time job to put on my orthopedic nurse's hat and take care of Ashley. I really wasn't fond of orthopedics when I was in nursing school, but it was what Ashley needed. She was in and out of The Children's Institute of Pittsburgh (TCI) (www.amazingkids.org) for about a year for rehabilitation. Sadly, we spent Christmas Eve and Christmas Day of 2003 at TCI. It was the toughest holiday I've ever lived through.

Ashley went back to school in February 2004 but still could not put any pressure on her legs. I would drive her in the morning, put her in a wheelchair, and wheel her into school. Her teachers were unbelievably supportive. I would go to work until about 3 pm and then go back to the school to pick her up. We then would go to rehabilitation for several hours. It was a very hectic schedule, and I was exhausted.

Ashley had to learn how to walk all over again. Her goal was to get back to cheering, so some of her rehabilitation involved exercises to strengthen the muscles she needed for all of her stunts. I coached her in cheering for a midget football team for two years as she regained her strength and tumbling skills. She also belonged to various competitive cheerleading organizations. We went to competitions in Pittsburgh; Columbus, Ohio; Washington, DC; and Virginia Beach, Virginia. She even cheered at a national competition in Orlando, Florida, in 2011. It was like the Super Bowl for cheerleaders! I went with her and we had a wonderful time. Around the same time, I had started my job at ONS and was supposed to attend our annual conference. I explained to my chief executive officer (CEO) that I was already committed to the Florida gig with my daughter (e.g., plane tickets bought, hotel deposit paid, uniform purchased) and could not get my money back. She was surprised yet was very supportive. Ashley was impressed that I chose her over my job. That's what we do. "Family First."

Patrick was 17 and a senior in high school when Amanda died. He was 19 and in his second year of college at Indiana University of Pennsylvania (IUP) when his dad died. When an IUP police officer knocked on his apartment door on the night of the crash, he thought he was being busted for underage drinking. Instead, a cab was waiting to drive Patrick 90 minutes to CHP. All he knew was that Ashley and his dad were in a car crash. When he arrived, most of my family (who had arrived in the interim) scattered, as they were afraid he would be suspicious about his dad by looking at their tear-filled faces. After he saw Ashley and knew she was OK, I took him into a separate room and told him about his dad. It was the most awful thing I ever had to do. We both cried at another incredible loss in our nuclear family.

After the holidays, he went back to IUP. However, he just couldn't concentrate on anything but his father's death, so he quit school and came home to help me take care of Ashley. He was a tremendous help.

He lost his mojo for school and waited several years to reconsider college. In 2012, he enrolled at Duquesne University in Pittsburgh, partially because that's where his dad went. He also started to volunteer at the Highmark Caring Place as a facilitator for kids who had experienced loss in their families. I think he was able to come to terms with Amanda's and Pat's deaths as he helped other children face the deaths of their loved ones. He has been there for about five years and has received several awards.

My Family Grows

I met my third and current husband Rulison (Hipp) Evans many years ago, as our families lived in the same borough. We got married on September 8, 2007.

My husband died in 2003; Hipp's wife died in 2006 from heart failure. They both were 42 years old.

I became a stepmom when Hipp and I got married. His daughter, Ashley Marie Evans, and my daughter, Ashley Marie Wertz, had been friends since the second grade. They cheered together and did lots of other things that best friends do. As kids, the two Ashleys had many sleepovers. When they stayed at my house, we would all snuggle together and talk about boys!

Ashley E. went on to graduate from IUP with a bachelor's degree in sports management. She is working for a gym in the Pittsburgh area and considering getting her master's degree.

I see her as another daughter and love her dearly.

In fact, it was through our children that my relationship with Hipp really developed. As we were shuttling kids back and forth to football games and other activities, we became good friends. Through time, Hipp and I grew closer and closer.

We blended our families by moving into a new house in the same area. It was a necessary move, as my kids did not want to live at his house and did not want him living in "Dad's house." It was tough for several years, as the kids had trouble adjusting. Even though we were all living together, it was difficult. Eventually, they all came around after we had been together about five years.

We still are doing very well today.

My Career

My career spanned from the early 1980s into the 21st century. Once I finished high school, I went to a secretarial school in downtown Pittsburgh. I completed the school's 18-month course, worked for several cardiovascular surgeons as a medical assistant and transcriptionist for a few years, and then started nursing school at the St. Francis General Hospital School of Nursing in August 1978, receiving an associate degree in nursing in 1980. I then worked in the CVICU for four years at the same hospital where I went to nursing school.

After working in the CVICU, I moved to Allegheny General Hospital in Pittsburgh in 1984. I created their Office of Prehospital Care and became the department's manager. During this time, I also was a flight nurse for a few years. I gave up flight duties when I decided to go back to school to get my BSN.

This process was a bit of a nightmare. I was a wife with a very supportive RN husband, took care of three kids (including one with special needs), and also had a full-time management job. I honestly don't know how I did it with all of those responsibilities. I received my BSN in 1993 from Carlow University in Pittsburgh then went straight into a master's program at Carnegie Mellon University.

Along the way, I wrote articles and book chapters, served as a book editor, and published a pediatric book in 2001 called *Emergency Care of Children*. A link to the book is on my website (www .panda-llc.com).

After 11 years at Allegheny General Hospital, I was laid off as part of a management reorganization in February 1995. I had a decent severance package, which enabled me to concentrate on school without working full time. When the severance ran out, I started working part time as a staff nurse in the ED at Sewickley Valley Hospital. Once I finished my master's degree in public management, I left the ED and started my executive career.

I moved into a physician practice as an executive director for a large cardiac group. I left there when a pediatric opportunity presented itself. I moved into this large pediatric practice (with 20 pediatricians and specialists) as its first executive director, eventually becoming its CEO. After 10 years, I left this group and started my own consulting business, PANDA and Associates, LLC.

In 2008, I started working on my PhD at Capella University through an online program. I attended all three colloquia throughout my time there and graduated with distinction in August 2013 with a PhD. It took five years but was so worth the investment of time and money. My dissertation was *Understanding Productivity and Technostress for Oncology Nurses Using an Electronic Health Record (EHR) to Increase Safety, Quality, and Effectiveness of Care for Patients With Cancer.*

The last stop of my career was at ONS in April 2011. At ONS, I served as the executive director of Professional Practice and Programs. It was a great role. I was leading staff, traveling to the capital, teaching, giving presentations, working on great projects, and going to many other places as an ONS representative.

I loved my job at ONS and all the opportunities it provided. I retired in January 2016. It was one of the hardest decisions of my life. I was working only two days a week but struggled to make it through those days. I began to realize that I would not be able to go back to a full-time job. I talked with several good friends and mentors to get additional pros and cons. Because I was no longer an executive, I felt like I was not doing anything meaningful. If my life was limited, I wanted to spend more time with my family and do things that made a difference.

My last day was January 28. The company gave me a retirement party in February. I didn't realize I had such an impact on so many people and was very pleased to spend those hours with everyone. I miss the work, yet not having a major "to-do" list really helped my fatigue. I have three writing projects in the pipeline that I can work on whenever I feel up to it.

My Fight Continues

I continue to take an oral chemotherapy med (Xeloda®) for one week on and one week off. The week that I am "on" is usually filled with side effects. I start to heal the week I am off but then go back on the drug just when I am feeling better. My oncologist said I may be on this routine for the rest of my life. As long as this med keeps the cancer from growing, I will continue to take it no matter how annoying the side effects.

At this stage, I'm really not the same person that I was before the current liver metastasis. Instead, I have to focus on doctor's appointments, medications, changes in meds, co-pays (Xeloda is $2,150 per refill), working with my local pharmacy, my emotional status, overwhelming fatigue, my life expectancy, and keeping up a good front for my kids. That doesn't even include fighting with my insurance company, especially when they decide an important test my doctor ordered is not covered. That process is very stressful and easily could lead to a whole other book!

I hope you enjoy reading about my experiences. I hope it will help you to be more aware of what patients and nurses go through every day, especially when those nurses are taking care of patients receiving chemotherapy. As nurses, our goal always has been to help provide the highest quality of care for patients with cancer. I hope this book gives you a glimpse into that world.

Anne's Reflection

When Liz asked me to help her with this book, my first instinct was to decline. I am a solitary writer and set deadlines for myself that most people find unrealistic to adhere to in a writing partnership. But it was Liz who asked, and anyone who has met Liz knows that she is hard to say no to. Not because she is demanding or bossy, but because she is so engaging and friendly and downright nice. To say no to her would be the wrong thing to do—almost impossible. So, I said yes.

Over the year that we wrote this book together, I learned more about Liz, especially the grit and grace she has shown in her journey. Liz is a strong woman, a survivor of not only cancer, but personal tragedy the likes of which most of us will thankfully never know.

If one would meet her in person, none of this would be noticeable. She reminds me a little of Tigger in Winnie the Pooh—energetic, enthusiastic, curious, cheerful, confident, bouncy. I felt connected to her from the moment we first met. In telling her story, Liz let me into her deepest, most private thoughts. She will do the same for you, the reader.

What we see in the media about cancer often is glorified and sanitized and usually has a happy ending. After all, that is what sells magazines and advertising space. The reality of cancer, especially metastatic cancer, is something else entirely.

I have learned a lot from writing the evidence-based commentary to Liz's experiences. I am the daughter of a two-time survivor of breast cancer, and I often wonder when it will happen to me. As an oncology nurse and an editor of the *Oncology Nursing Forum*, I know a thing or two about breast cancer. In reviewing the literature for this book, I learned even more.

But the lessons I've learned from Liz cannot be found in any journal or textbook. I will carry them in my heart and into my life.

Chapter 1.
The Cancer Diagnosis

Today is my youngest daughter Ashley W.'s 17th birthday. Today is the day I hear those words every woman dreads . . . "You have breast cancer."

I talked to Carol at the oncologist's office at around 9:30 am. She is the oncology nurse who told me the news by phone (as I requested when I was in the office). She said I have infiltrating lobular cancer, the second most common type of breast cancer. All I could say was, "Oh shit." I joked with her about not saying the "F" word. She told me a lot of people say it. I'm sure it will come out of my mouth sooner or later. She also told me that my tumor is estrogen receptor positive (ER+), meaning the circulating estrogen in my body is feeding the tumor.

Despite being the second most common form of breast cancer, invasive or infiltrating lobular carcinoma occurs in only 10%–15% of women with breast cancer. It often is multifocal with irregular borders and feels hard to palpation. The hormonal status of the tumor also is very important; Liz's tumor was ER+, meaning the tumor needs estrogen to grow. This is a good sign, as these types of tumors usually are sensitive to medications that reduce the amount of estrogen in the blood, a hallmark of adjuvant endocrine treatment with drugs such as tamoxifen and/or aromatase inhibitors (see pp. 46–47) (Yackzan, 2011).

It doesn't really feel like I have a tumor. There were tiny calcifications on the mammogram I had on August 20 (my husband's birthday) that were not there last year. I have these mammograms done religiously every year. I didn't feel anything, and you could barely see anything on the film. The physician I see every 6–12 months for this testing saved my life by seeing these tiny dots. I plan to send her a thank-you card (which I did).

Screening mammography is used in healthy women with no family history of cancer as part of routine preventive health care. The frequency of these mammograms is a controversial topic. Recent recommendations from the U.S. Preventive Services Task Force (2016) state that mammogram screening every two years in women aged 40–49 should be done based on an individual woman's values and circumstances (that is, not routinely). For women aged 50–74, screening should be done every two years; it is this age group that sees the maximum benefit from screening in terms of mortality. Harms associated with screening exist, including psychological effects, increased imaging and biopsies, high false-positive results, and unnecessary treatment and radiation exposure (U.S. Preventive Services Task Force, 2016). Reducing the frequency of mammograms to every two years decreases these harms by half while retaining the benefits of annual screening.

The American Cancer Society (n.d.) recommends a slightly different schedule for screening, with yearly mammograms beginning at age 45, then reducing in frequency to every other year at age 55 or annually depending on individual preference.

Many women and healthcare providers question these recommendations. Changes in breast tissue can happen in the intervals between mammograms, as Liz experienced. Women may be fearful that a longer interval between screenings may result in a bigger tumor and/or a later stage at diagnosis; however, for some women, lengthening the time between mammograms appears to make little difference in outcome and may lessen the anxiety of having the screening test.

The other kind of mammogram is called a diagnostic mammogram. This essentially is the same technology, but the images are viewed in real time. A radiologist will ask for additional images if something abnormal is seen. This may result in a biopsy from a concerning area of breast tissue, which is then examined by a pathologist. A biopsy is a definitive test for breast cancer, confirming or excluding its presence.

I came home and talked to Hipp (my husband) and Patty (my sister). I got a bit tearful as I was apologizing to my husband for "defective merchandise." We have been married for only two years. He told me not to be ridiculous. My sister and I ended up laughing, as I was really making fun of myself. I'm going to rely on these two quite a bit. I have so many things planned for September and October—two conferences, two classes at school, etc. I decided not to cancel or rearrange anything today because I don't really know enough details yet of what will happen to me. I put on a happy face and went to lunch with Ashley W. (my biological daughter, as she calls herself), Ashley E. (my stepdaughter), and a bunch of their friends to celebrate Ashley W.'s birthday. It actually was fun, and I did all I could to block the news out of my brain.

I told Patrick (my son) when he got home from work. As my oldest child, he deserved to know first. I explained to him that I would not be telling the Ashleys for a few more days. Between Ashley W.'s birthday today and the first day of school tomorrow, I did not want to cause them any more stress.

FYI—I have called my breasts "the girls" ever since I can remember. I named them Thelma and Louise (from the movie). Thelma, on the right, is the bad one (where the cancer is located). Louise is on the left. I always joke around about them with the Ashleys and their friends. I even asked my friend Monica how her new "girls" were when I saw her on August 9, as she just had reconstructive surgery after going through this same nightmare.

September 3, 2009

I went to the breast center in my neighborhood, which is part of a university and multihospital organization, to get a breast MRI (actually, both breasts). I saw the words on my forms, and it started to sink in . . . "Newly Diagnosed Breast CA." It started to feel much more real.

A magnetic resonance imaging (MRI) study is a highly sensitive scan used (in addition to traditional mammography) to identify physical characteristics of a tumor. It has a higher rate of false-positive results and generally is not used as a screening test for breast cancer. It is used in women with newly diagnosed, biopsy-proven breast cancer to check if there are other small tumors in the breast and/or if the contralateral breast is cancer-free.

This wonderful nurse, Carol, came out to meet me. She is the woman who gave me the news yesterday over the phone. She almost started to cry. She gave me a big hug and then handed me this whole packet of information to read. Wow. It *is* real.

I then met Mel, the MRI technician. She started an IV and ushered me back to the room. When she put in the needle, it really hurt. I asked her, "Was that a 12-gauge?" (For all of you nonmedical people, this is a larger needle used for trauma patients.) She said, "No, it's only a 20-gauge (which is small)." Holy crap. If a 20-gauge needle hurt, what the hell am I going to do about real pain? I hate to be in any kind of pain!

I had to lie on my stomach with "the girls" hanging down through two separate holes. It actually was pretty funny, and I joked around with Mel about it. I quickly saw that I will lose any of my modesty. After about 40 minutes of very loud banging noises, I was all done and had one hell of a headache. I joked around some more about the headache and told Mel she will be in the book I plan to write. After I was dressed, I saw Dr. G. out in the hallway. She was jogging outside between appointments and was all sweaty. She came over and gave me a big hug. I didn't even mind the sweat. She was the physician who did the biopsy on August 28. She said she was so shocked that the pathology report came back showing cancer. Me too.

Waiting for the results of diagnostic testing is highly anxiety provoking and distressing (Montgomery & McCrone, 2010), even with an understanding of the medical issues, as Liz has. Anxiety exists during the testing phase of the diagnostic journey and is decreased only by a benign result. If results show that the person has cancer, anxiety remains high, no matter how quickly the process unfolds (Brocken, Prins, Dekhuijzen, & van der Heijden, 2012). Distress is very common in women newly diagnosed with breast cancer. In one study, 77% of women studied reported distress, manifesting as worry and nervousness (Mertz et al., 2012).

Labor Day weekend, 2009

We had my mom (Helen), my dad (Bill), my brother (Charlie), and some friends over this weekend. We swam, cooked out, and had a great bonfire on Sunday evening. The weather sucked all day Monday (rain), so we stayed inside. I played cards with my mom, which was fun and reminded me of much younger days! Having all of us together was very encouraging for me. Even though I was so afraid to have any surgery, it was reassuring to know that my family was going to help me however they could. I still am very frightened and unsure about what happens next. Will I need chemotherapy? Will I lose my hair? What are my chances for survival?

Coping after a diagnosis of cancer has been widely studied. How a woman copes in the initial days and weeks after hearing the words "you have cancer" may affect her ultimate survival. Watson, Homewood, and Haviland (2012) concluded that poor coping may lead to a poor outcome. The converse, however, does not apply; good coping does not mean better survival. The authors concluded that poor coping is associated with depression, sleep and appetite disturbances, unhealthy lifestyles, and an inability to ask for and access help—all of which may contribute to poor outcomes.

Other researchers have found that a sense of personal control is a positive factor (Henselmans et al., 2010); women who have a greater sense of control in their lives are more engaged in their social lives during active treatment, helping them to control anxiety. Controlling anxiety through distraction and by accessing social support when necessary may lead to better long-term outcomes. How a woman initially reacts to a diagnosis may influence her well-being as many as three years later (Hack & Degner, 2004). These researchers found that women who respond to a breast cancer diagnosis with passive acceptance and a resigned outlook have poorer long-term adjustment.

One of the critical tasks for women after a cancer diagnosis is maintaining a sense of self-integrity after the shock and threat to life (Lally, 2010). This is theorized to happen

through a process of acclimating to the diagnosis by survey-
ing the situation, taking action, and emerging as a new person, stronger than before.

September 8, 2009

Today is my second wedding anniversary. My husband has been
terrific so far with this mess. I know that God brought him to me in
preparation for this latest battle. I really am blessed, even with this
latest challenge. God must have other plans for me. Today, I thought
a lot about my kids and my husband. As a blended family, we still
are working through some issues. I can't imagine the four of them
(my two children, my husband, and his daughter) trying to get along
without me there as the peacemaker. It was a very scary feeling and
one that I quickly dismissed.

The support of a spouse and other family members is very
important during the diagnostic phase and through active
treatment. Most spouses are supportive, but evidence exists
that conflict can arise, particularly as treatment continues over
months. In one study (Sprung, Janotha, & Steckel, 2011), some
spouses became abusive and controlling; however, this may
have been reflective of their usual personality traits. *Couples
coping* is based on how each member appraises the threat
from the cancer, how they communicate their fears, and how
they create meaning from the experience. Of particular interest from this study was that some participants felt that their
healthcare providers missed opportunities to address stress
within their relationships. This occurred when professionals
either ignored statements from the patient or did not offer
support to the partner/spouse, even when it was disclosed
that the partner was experiencing stress. Evidence exists of

interdependence of patient and partner distress as they adjust to the diagnosis, particularly in physical symptoms such as loss of appetite and nausea (Segrin & Badger, 2014).

Family members may have a variety of unmet needs, including their own emotional response to the diagnosis and the accompanying distress. They may need help with accessing information about the cancer, the treatment options, and what to expect (Schmid-Büchi, van den Borne, Dassen, & Halfens, 2011).

September 10, 2009

I'm finding it very hard to concentrate today, as the thought of cancer fills my mind. In 2008, I started an online program to get my doctorate. Right now, I have two weeks' worth of homework due by Sunday night. I just can't get into it. Instead, I am doing some research on breast cancer.

September 10 was supposed to be exciting, as it's the date of the first Steelers home game since their sixth Super Bowl win in February 2009. Instead, it now has more personal meaning as "the day before I see the surgeon." However, I still plan to enjoy the Steelers game tonight and will try to worry about that other "stuff" tomorrow.

GO STEELERS! Trash those Titans!

September 11, 2009

Well, first, say some prayers for all of the victims and their families from that tragedy eight years ago today. I can't believe so much time has elapsed. Second, I saw the surgeon today. I really liked her and feel SO much better after we talked. I will be having a lumpectomy done on September 29, at which time they also will remove some of my lymph nodes. They will test the nodes for cancer, and my ongoing treatment will be based on whatever they find. I will need at least radiation and have two options. One is called MammoSite (who comes up with these names?) and is considered targeted radiation therapy. The surgeon puts this catheter with a balloon on it into the cavity left after the lumpectomy. I would then go twice a day, six hours apart, for five days to have radiation seeds put into the balloon. The advantage to this method is that it is over in five days and it only radiates the area where the cancer cells were originally located. The second option is external radiation, once per day, five days per week, for about six weeks.

Women consider a number of factors when making a decision about treatment, including what they believe will be the best treatment for them, what they know about other women who have been treated, and any information that they have been provided. Other factors include their age, where they live, accessibility to centers that offer their treatment, and their family history. Ultimately, the woman's autonomy is the deciding factor in making a treatment decision (Bride et al., 2013). Hack and Degner (2004) suggest that women involved in their treatment decision experience less regret later on and have better quality of life and social and physical functioning than those who take a more passive role in their treatment decisions. Most women involved in making a treatment decision are satisfied with their treatment; those not involved tend to be less satisfied (Budden, Hayes, & Buettner, 2014).

At this stage, I won't know anything about needing chemotherapy until the pathology results are back after the surgery. That process takes about four working days. I was told that I will need to take tamoxifen (or another drug if I am postmenopausal) after all of the radiation/chemotherapy is completed. I will need to stay on it for five years.

Once the tumor has been removed, the pathology will be determined and if (like most breast cancers) it is hormone dependent (estrogen and/or progesterone), adjuvant therapy will be recommended. Depending on the menopausal status of the woman, different types of treatment are prescribed. Tamoxifen is a selective estrogen receptor modulator (SERM), usually prescribed for women who are premenopausal, and is taken for five years after primary treatment.

I guess I feel like there is more of a plan at this point. Things are not so "up in the air" anymore. I know what at least some of the process will be. That is a much better feeling. Now I have to wait 18 days until the next step, but at least I know what it will be.

So, I'm off to live life for two weeks before I need to slow down for a bit. I will finish the requirements for the two classes I am taking and start reading for the next ones. My husband and I may even try to get away for a few days to spend some uninterrupted time together.

All those prayers are helping. Keep them coming!

September 14, 2009

Hi, everyone! Well, today is a very positive day. The sun is shining, the sky is blue, and I am fully alive!

Even more exciting is my new website. Please check it out at www.panda-llc.com. A fellow by the name of T.J. put it all together and did an amazing job. I am so proud of what he was able to do with the information I gave to him.

Make sure you check out the "About Amanda" and "Organ Donation Saves Lives" icons on the upper-right corner. Those pages are terrific, if I do say so myself.

Trying to keep the positive vibes going . . .

September 28, 2009
Almost surgery day!

Well, tomorrow is the big day. I have to be at the hospital at 6:30 am and the radiology suite by 7 am. They will insert a wire into my breast so the surgeon knows where to go. I then will go to the operating room (OR), where surgery is scheduled for 8:30 am.

My husband and my sister will be at the hospital with me. I am allowed to come home after everything is over and when I am awake. Patty will post something the afternoon of to let everyone know how things went.

I won't know the specific stage of the cancer until the final pathology report. My first postoperative visit is on October 5, at which time the reports will be back and we will discuss the next steps.

I am off to the girls' high school to do concession stand duty, one of the pleasures of being a cheerleading mom! I actually enjoy doing it. Then, tonight, I plan to watch a bunch of comedies to get my positive hormones going.

Talk to you all after the surgery. Keep those prayers coming for me!

September 29, 2009
Update on Liz's surgery

This is Patty, Liz's sister, and I wanted to let all of you know her surgery went really well today. Four lymph nodes were removed, and preliminary results showed they were free of any cancer cells. The mass also was removed with no complications. Further tests will be done on the nodes and mass, with results to be presented to Liz and her husband at her next appointment on Monday, October 5. Everyone is very positive with the surgery and the results so far. Her spirits were good and she now is home.

September 30, 2009

My first day as a survivor!

Well, I have been away from my computer less than 24 hours. Wow. I didn't think I would feel this good.

Hipp, Patty, and I were at the hospital at 6:30 am yesterday. My first trip was to the breast center radiology suite, where they injected a radioactive isotope into my breast. That one hurt. Then they injected some lidocaine (just a small pinch for a bunch of numbness—good tradeoff) and inserted a small guidewire into the area of the cancer. After more mammogram pictures (ouch) to confirm the placement and a hug from Dr. G., I went to the preoperative area. Robert, who was the facility's employee of the year, was my escort. Nothing but the best for me!

There, they asked me the same questions and started an IV. I was impressed with their level of safety! They all were very efficient and very caring. I am such a warm and fuzzy person that I loved the hugs and the kindness. I have known many nurses in my career that were pretty cranky on the job. None of them worked here—thank goodness.

The comfort that the staff, in particular the nurses, provided Liz was extremely important. As a nurse herself, Liz no doubt was judging their actions by her standards. Not all nurses hug their patients, but these nurses seemed to know what Liz needed. Their kindness and physical demonstrations of support helped her at a time of extreme anxiety. Patients place a great deal of importance on the technical and/or clinical expertise of the nurse because this is what makes them feel safe. While the caring nature of the nurse is important, it is safety that builds trust (Wiechula et al., 2016).

Hipp and Patty then came back for some entertainment. My friend Monica, who is a two-time breast cancer survivor, made me this beautiful heart pillow (lime green and pink with butterflies—it was perfect). Patty was telling everyone she had a heart-on. She had everyone laughing, which was a great distraction. I love that girl!

The nurse let me walk into the OR. That was crazy. I asked her if I would be walking out and she said, "Not likely." Ha ha! They had this heated, inflatable thing on the OR table that was wonderfully warm. I got the top line of service! However, the electrocardiogram pads were pretty chilly. I lay down and of course was talking my head off. There's a surprise! The nurse anesthetist said, "I'm going to give you a little midazolam," instead of saying, "Please stop talking!"

I chatted for a few more minutes and then said, "Did you give me the midazolam?"

"Yep," she said. And that was it.

The next thing I knew, I was waking up and asking if it was all over. After some Diet Pepsi and some crackers, Hipp and Patty came into the room. By that time, I was awake and asking about the lymph nodes. They were negative at first peek! My prayers (and all of yours) were answered here. They took only four nodes out, so I did not have a drain in place. Yippee!

Sentinel lymph node biopsy is the standard of care in assessing whether breast cancer has spread outside of the breast tissue into the axillary lymph nodes. It replaced the axillary lymph node dissection associated with the development of lymphedema and injuries to the shoulder. Sentinel lymph node biopsy is based on the theory that the breast is drained by axillary lymph nodes in an orderly fashion and,

> if the sentinel lymph node is cancer-free, it is unlikely that
> other lymph nodes are affected, making spread beyond the
> breast unlikely (Manca et al., 2015).

Around noon, the nurse said I was ready to go home. I put all my Steelers clothes back on (everyone commented on them) and walked to the car. I pretty much slept all afternoon. Hipp made me tea and something to eat and generally took really great care of me. For a nonmedical guy, he's not too shabby! Patty went home because she had been up since 4 am.

I am amazed at how good I feel. I can lift my arm, which means I can do my own hair. Another yippee!

I slept fairly well last night yet was up at 5 am—time to take a pain pill (oxycodone). I am much sorer today but nothing unbearable. The worst part is the itching from the pain medicine, for which I am taking diphenhydramine. When the nurse calls today, I'll see about switching to another pain med because of the itching.

Well, the drugs are starting to take effect, so I am going to lie back down and rest. Keep those kind thoughts and prayers coming. They are helping.

October 2, 2009

Another bump in the road . . .

I just talked with the surgeon. She told me that all of the lymph nodes were negative, which is great news. She also told me that not all of the margins they removed around the original cancer area were clean. I see her Monday morning for a follow-up visit. I then will have more surgery on Tuesday afternoon to remove a larger area of tissue. The second surgery can be done using conscious sedation. If they cannot get all of the margins clean with this second surgery, I will have to have a mastectomy.

I am incredibly grateful that the nodes did not show any signs of cancer. However, I am in shock that there still is more in there that she didn't get the first time around. I feel kind of numb right now.

If the surgical margins are not clear of cancer cells, a woman may need another surgery to make sure that all the cancer has been removed; this is a risk of breast-conserving surgery (lumpectomy) (Lyle et al., 2016). This is distressing for women and has cosmetic, financial, and emotional side effects (Merrill et al., 2016).

October 5, 2009
Surgeon's visit today

I saw the surgeon this morning, and we discussed the next steps. She told me she was surprised that she didn't get everything during the first surgery, but invasive lobular cancer can be very tricky. She is not sure yet if I will need chemotherapy.

I'm scheduled for another surgery tomorrow at 2:30 pm. She will remove more tissue and send it to the laboratory. She should have the results back from pathology by Thursday or Friday. If the margins still are not clean, I will need a mastectomy.

The nurse gave me a copy of the pathology report. When I left the office, I sat in the car, read it, and cried. It all is starting to sink in that I really have this awful disease and that it is not going to be quite so simple to get rid of it.

I am pretty discouraged at this moment and finished off the rest of the chocolate chip cookies that my friend Stephanie baked for me. Thank you, Stephanie! They were wonderful.

I am tempted to just go back to bed and lie there until tomorrow around noon. However, I start two new classes today. Instead, I am going to sit outside in the sunshine and read about financial management. How's that for a great distraction?

Thank you also to my friend Sandy for her prayer today. She reminded me that God is in control and I have to have faith. I'm really trying. Please keep those prayers coming, as I am showing some weakness here.

Distress can occur at any stage of the cancer journey. While it is common at the time of diagnosis, dealing with it then does not mean that it will not reoccur, especially around the time when the patient moves from active treatment into recovery and the survivorship phase. For Liz, learning that she would need additional surgery because the surgical margins weren't clear was extremely distressing. This has been shown in other studies, including one where anxiety was the dominant form of distress (Jørgensen, Garne, Søgaard, & Laursen, 2015). Women in this study were worried about recurrence, dying, losing confidence in the healthcare system, and the need for repeated tests.

Liz drew on her faith as a way of dealing with her distress. It has been shown that women who draw on their faith and see God as engaged in their life tend to cope better and, as a result, are less concerned about recurrence (Schreiber, 2011). Another study showed that women who participated in a spiritual therapy intervention had improved quality of life compared to those who had only standard care (Jafari et al., 2013). Conversely, McLaughlin et al. (2013) found that while giving over control to God can lower levels of worry about breast cancer, it also can lead to a more passive coping that may result in lower quality of life.

October 6, 2009

Liz's surgery went well today. She is quite sore but is home resting. Hopefully, we will know the results by Monday and the next steps. I am sure she will be posting soon. Until then, keep her in your thoughts and prayers.

—Patty

October 8, 2009
Surgery #2

Well, this time around was a bit rougher than surgery #1. I was very emotional and was crying during radiology. They had to insert a wire into my breast while doing a mammogram. The squeezing part was very painful, especially with a fresh surgical site!

Getting to the OR (and the drugs) was the easiest part. I woke up without any problem. Dr. M., the surgeon, thinks she got everything. We hopefully will know by Friday what the pathology report shows. I then see her in the office on Monday, October 12.

I am much more tired after this surgery. I literally have been in bed until almost noon both days and then just lying around watching TV. I feel lazy, yet I just don't feel like doing anything else. I am listening to my body.

My biggest disappointment right now is that I won't be able to attend the Medical Group Management Association (MGMA) national conference. I am so incredibly sad that I will not get to see everyone and participate in the meetings. This year's conference would have been my 13th in a row. I know I am doing the right thing by staying home, but I really feel bad about not being there.

Keep those positive thoughts and prayers coming. I still need them. Hugs to all of you for standing beside me in this journey.

October 9, 2009
Thelma gets to stay!

Carol from Dr. M.'s office called me this morning with good news. The pathology report showed that the margins were clear this time, so Thelma gets to stay with me! Boy, is she happy about that! For those of you who have no idea what I am talking about, NO MASTECTOMY!

I see Dr. M. on Monday, October 12, at which time we will talk about the next steps. Carol said I will probably need radiation to the entire breast, instead of just the local, internal option. They will set up visits to the medical and radiation oncologists.

> Lumpectomy and radiation is one treatment option available to women; it is a breast-conserving treatment, as it does not involve removal of the entire breast (as in a mastectomy). It has been shown to have similar outcomes to mastectomy, with fewer postsurgical complications and side effects. Radiation is necessary after the lumpectomy to ensure survival rates equal to a mastectomy (Yackzan & Hatch, 2011).

Thank you for your prayers, your cards, and your kind words of encouragement. This road is still going to be tough, but I feel a renewed energy from the news today. I have been praying for strength to handle whatever the news would be and have been thanking God all morning for the positive results! I feel stronger already!

So, it's time for me to get off my ass, quit feeling sorry for myself, and move on! I am listening to Keith Urban right now. "These are the days we will remember. Live them while you can. Go live your life." Amen, brother! I have an article to finish and a bunch of homework to get done. This weekend is homecoming at the high school, so I get to see my beautiful daughters all dressed up and enjoying their junior year. Life is good.

October 12, 2009
Another visit with the surgeon

I saw Dr. M. today for my second postoperative visit (related to the reexcision surgery on October 6). The incisions are healing well, and she is pleased with my recovery. She confirmed that the margins were clean and gave me a copy of the latest pathology report. I need to see her again in three months. Of course, I am their favorite patient!

They are making referrals to a medical oncologist and a radiation oncologist. I have to wait for the results of another test before I see either of them. The test is called an Oncotype DX, and it is run on the tissue removed from my breast. Once complete, it gives a score that gauges the potential for recurrence. They sent everything to a laboratory in California after the surgery, and results may be back by the 14th of this month. (That's Wednesday for those of you without a calendar immediately available.) If the score is 0 to 18, I won't need any chemotherapy. If the score is between 19 and 31, I will probably need chemotherapy. Anything greater than 31 is a definite. Dr. M. said that even if I need chemotherapy, I would need "only" four treatments—easy for her to say. If necessary, I would get the chemotherapy before any radiation therapy.

Oncotype DX is a genetic assay that allows for decisions to be made about the need for chemotherapy to prevent recurrence in women with breast cancer that has not spread to the lymph nodes (Nguyen et al., 2014). This test is widely used by oncologists to help them decide whether chemotherapy will be useful for a particular patient, and it may help patients understand why they are being offered additional treatment or not.

So, I have to wait for the results of this test before I know the next steps for treatment. The hardest parts are the uncertainty and feeling like I'm putting my life on hold. Oh well. I always have homework to finish to keep my mind off of the waiting.

It is extremely common for women with breast cancer to struggle with the uncertainty associated with the cancer itself and the trajectory that it will take. In addition, patients face a myriad of decisions that need to be made about treatment, going back to work, telling others about the cancer, etc. Waiting is difficult under any circumstances. Waiting to hear if chemotherapy is necessary is extremely challenging, given the understanding that chemotherapy takes place over months and has significant side effects.

October 15, 2009

17 is my lucky number!

I just talked with the surgeon's office. The Oncotype DX came back and was 17, which means NO CHEMOTHERAPY! THANK THE LORD! THANK YOU, THANK YOU, THANK YOU!

I also just talked with the medical oncologist's office. I will see Dr. O. (ha ha, I know what some of you are thinking—I do NOT need a doctor in that area!) on Monday morning at 11. I then see the radiation oncologist on Tuesday at 10 am.

I feel sooo much better. Now, I can stop sitting around feeling sorry for myself and get on with my life. Woo-hoo!

Because I get to keep my hair, I'm now calling to make an appointment to get my roots done.

October 16, 2009

Well, I went to the hairdresser today and came out feeling like a million bucks. No more roots! My hair had grown more than two inches since my last appointment in July. It even felt good to have her yanking at my hair as she was drying it. I am just so thankful to have all my hair and to be keeping it.

Hair loss is one of the major fears of women who need to have chemotherapy as part of their treatment for breast cancer. McGarvey, Baum, Pinkerton, and Rogers (2001) reported that this is the most traumatic side effect for women and that it added to the distress of the original diagnosis. It is no wonder that Liz was so elated that she did not need chemotherapy. Her response to what would be regarded as an ordinary experience for most women at the hairdresser is a reflection of her relief.

Tonight is a big football game at the high school. It is rainy/snowy, so it should be a blast to sit in that mess for three hours . . . NOT! That's OK, though; I still have my hair to get all wet and frizzy. I'll be doing it again on Sunday at the Steelers vs. Browns game (although I hear the rain/snow may subside by game time).

Enjoy the weekend, everyone. Hugs and kisses to you all!

Upcoming treatment

I spent the last three days going back and forth to an outpatient center at the hospital. The worst part was walking into an area with a big sign that said "Cancer Center." I couldn't believe that I was there for me. There were a bunch of people in the waiting room, and I found myself looking at everyone and thinking, *Are you here for treatment or waiting for someone?* There were a few people there with no hair, so I knew they were patients. That part was tough.

On Monday, I met with Dr. O. (ha ha), who is now my medical oncologist. The doc and the staff were very nice. They drew blood to send labs to check my menopause status. Dr. O. said I will probably start tamoxifen in the middle of the radiation treatments and then possibly change once they know my status.

Women who have hormone receptor-positive breast cancer are prescribed hormone-blocking medication after their initial treatment (surgery, radiation, and/or chemotherapy) to prevent a recurrence of the breast cancer.

Yesterday, I met with Dr. M. (not the same one from before!), who is now my radiation oncologist. She and her nurse were VERY nice and caring and answered all of my questions. I really didn't know squat about radiation, other than the safety article I read about radiation errors—scary. They explained the process and what I should expect. They also did some measurements and gave Thelma some very small tattoos to use for the radiation treatments. She wanted Steelers tattoos, but they weren't big enough (the tattoos, that is).

It is very important for the patient to be in the same position for every radiation treatment. The linear accelerator, the machine that generates the beams of radiation toward the area of the breast where the tumor was removed, is programmed very precisely, and the patient has to be in the same position to allow accuracy. To ensure

---

that this occurs, small tattoos are inked on the patient's skin. These are lined up with laser beams to confirm that the patient is in the right spot for the treatment. These tattoo marks usually are blue dots and not the Steelers tattoos that Liz wanted.

I have to have a total of 32 treatments. Twenty-five of them will be directed toward all of Thelma. I then will get seven boosters directly to the area where they removed the cancer. I will go five days per week for almost seven weeks. Dr. M. said the worst part is going to the hospital every day and working it into my schedule. The actual radiation process takes about 10 minutes.

I left the hospital and went to visit my parents, who live about 10 minutes away. My mom, dad, and I sat at the dining room table just chatting for a few hours. It was really quite nice. My dad told me I looked nice (must have noticed the newly colored hair).

Today, I was back at the hospital for a computed tomography (CT) scan of my chest. Dr. M. will review it and come up with what they call a rad or radiation plan. I will see her again in about a week to go over all of the details and confirm the measurements.

Yesterday was my nephew Eric's 21st birthday. I can't believe he is that old already. We are going to my sister's house tonight to celebrate. He was too busy the day before drinking with his buddies.

More to follow . . .

November 3, 2009
Radiation treatments

I went to the cancer center today to finalize plans for my radiation treatments. The technologist took a bunch of measurements and gave me two more tiny tattoos. I will start on Thursday and go each day at 10 am. My last treatment should be on December 23, just in time for Christmas. I asked a million questions, and the technologist explained everything to me. He was very sweet and quite patient with me. The last seven treatments will be "boosters" to what he called the tumor bed, where the actual cancer was removed.

The whole process seems quite surreal at this point. Physically, I feel so much better yet am nervous about all that radiation penetrating my body. However, this too shall pass as I get into the routine. The people there were very nice, which certainly decreased my anxiety. Even the fellas at the valet area were very kind. In fact, they were trying to barter with me for my Steelers jacket. I told them they could keep my car before I would give up that coat. My kids gave it to me for my 50th birthday—lots of sentimental value. I told them I'm waiting for the seventh Super Bowl to sew on two more patches.

OK, that's it for now. Keep those prayers coming. They are working!

It is not at all unusual for someone with cancer, even a nurse such as Liz, to be nervous about having treatment. There is so much that is not known for patients—what it will feel like, how they will respond, what side effects will happen and when, and how this will affect their quality of life. While educating oneself may be helpful to a patient, the unknown continues to be anxiety provoking. It is not just the not knowing what will happen that is bothersome; it also is not knowing how you will react to the treatment, to any pain, to the side effects, etc. Even for a nurse, Liz is stepping into a world that she doesn't know much about, which is scary. Perhaps it is because she knows about the dangers of radiation that she is afraid.

November 9, 2009
Day 3 of radiation treatments

I started radiation treatments last Thursday, which was very psychologically traumatizing for me. I didn't feel anything yet was really spooked by the whole thing. As a nurse, I always was taught to get out of the patient room during a portable x-ray and to stay away from radiation. Now, I was actively being radiated, which really freaked me out. I almost threw up on the drive home. After a few hours, I got my head together. I also talked with another friend of mine, who is getting radiation treatments at the same place. That conversation was very helpful.

This is an example of how a nurse becoming a patient is not always an easy transition to make. All healthcare providers are taught to avoid exposure to all forms of radiation during their daily work; ongoing exposure to various sources of radiation during the average nursing career is not insignificant. Now, Liz has to put herself directly in the line of radiation, contradicting everything she has been taught over her career. No wonder she had the reaction she did!

Today, I went to the hospital for my third radiation treatment. Now I count the seconds when the buzzer is going off—24 seconds from one direction and 26 seconds from the other. The staff is very nice, and I even met some older people that lived on the same street where I grew up! Pretty amazing! It's kind of like the 10 am coffee klatch, with all of us sitting around chatting until it is our turn.

Today also is the eighth anniversary of Amanda's death. I went to her grave after the treatment and, for the first time, imagined my own headstone next to hers. Again, spooky. I thought about Ashley and Patrick coming to visit all three of us—Pat, Amanda, and me. I have since blocked the thought out of my mind. Positive things happen to positive thinkers!

Positive thinking is defined as an intentional coping style that stresses positive thoughts and suppresses negative thoughts (Ruthig, Holfeld, & Hanson, 2012). It is associated with having a fighting spirit in the face of cancer. Many people with cancer think that they have to be positive in order to get through the experience. However, there are some negative aspects to this; patients may place a burden on themselves by thinking positively and thinking they control something that, in many ways, is not in their control (Ruthig & Holfeld, 2016). Wilkinson and Kitzinger (2000) suggest that positive thinking is not really a cognitive coping style but a widely used idiom; there is social pressure for people with cancer to say that they are thinking positively, while what positive thinking really means is vague.

This is the memorial that I had printed in the *Pittsburgh Post-Gazette* today:

Amanda Elizabeth Wertz

June 11, 1987 to November 9, 2001

Today marks eight long years since we have seen your beautiful face. Earlier this year, I created a consulting company and named it after you, Amanda Panda. The website includes several pages about you with links to many wonderful organizations (www.panda-llc.com). My work on patient safety and quality is an ongoing tribute to you.

In July, we met the beautiful young woman, Dayna, who lives today because of her transplant on November 10, 2001. It is your liver that gave her a second chance at life. I could feel your love when she hugged me for the first time! She is staying in the Pittsburgh area while she goes to school so we get to see her once in a while. Her family is terrific. In fact, her younger sister's birthday is today. Happy birthday, Emily! Our relationship with Dayna and her family has helped to ease the pain of your loss. We all continue to carry on your memory and are thankful for the 14 years you were with us.

We love you and miss you, pretty girl.

Mom, Patrick, and Ashley

Give Daddy a kiss and hug from all of us!

Below is a link to some wonderful memories of Amanda.

www.panda-llc.com/amanda.html

December 14, 2009
25 down!

Well, today marked my 25th radiation treatment. Wow. I can't believe that many have gone by already. Tomorrow, I start the booster doses that are aimed specifically at the area where the tumor was (instead of my entire breast). Thank goodness, because Thelma is burnt to a crisp at this point. Yowsa!

Besides my skin being incredibly itchy and peeling (I know, not a very nice picture in your mind right now), I am much more tired. I feel like I could sleep all day, yet I toss and turn when I finally go to bed. I saw the physician today, and she recommended that I take a pain pill before bed to help with the discomfort. OK, doctor's orders!

Skin damage over an area that has been exposed to radiation is not uncommon (Shigematsu et al., 2006). Inflammation of the skin typically occurs within a week or two from the start of treatment and persists for some time, depending on the severity of the damage. As reported by Ferraro and Catanzaro (2011), radiation damage is characterized by four stages. Stage 1 is the mildest, with some redness and skin peeling similar to a sunburn. Stages 2–4 include increasing damage, with ulceration as the most serious manifestation.

Patients are educated about preventing and managing skin damage during and after radiation therapy. Using a gentle soap and patting dry (rather than rubbing) after bathing is an important preventive measure. Radiation therapists and nurses are trained to treat radiation damage and give instructions to patients specific to the symptoms experienced.

Fatigue often appears around the third week of treatment and persists for some time after the end of treatment. Patients often need more sleep than usual. It is recommended that they have periods of rest during the day and prioritize their activities. Light physical activity can help to decrease fatigue, even though patients may feel too tired to exercise. Most women find they are back to their usual energy levels three months after radiation therapy is completed.

I did get a bit of Christmas shopping done on Sunday because there was no Steelers game. We had a field day at Dick's Sporting Goods, so I think the kids are done. My son just wants money to go on a ski trip, but I did get him some new ski socks to help keep his little piggies warm. Last week was very hectic, yet I finished a 60-page chapter on patient safety for oncology nurses and turned in my two papers (about another 50 pages) for school. I checked today and saw that I got an "A" in one class (I know; overachiever!). The other grade is not posted yet. I plan to order my books now for next semester to get a head start on the reading.

Well, that's it for now. I hope all of you are enjoying the season and aren't too crazy yet. I am going to see my girlfriends tonight, as we have our holiday get-together.

<u>December 23, 2009</u>

I finished my last radiation treatment today. It felt great to be done after so many trips to the cancer center.

The end of treatment comes as a relief for some and a challenge for others. It is a source of various emotions, not all of which are positive. Many patients find transitioning out of active treatment to be difficult. For months or even years, the person has been a "patient" and under the care and scrutiny of a treatment team. This affords some with a sense of safety and protection. Moving away from the intensity of acute treatment leaves some feeling vulnerable. Ending active treatment means moving away from the "fighting" phase to a more subtle monitoring phase. This can be scary for some. It also means the end of daily or weekly trips to the cancer center or hospital. This can be a relief, but it also can mean the loss of contact with other patients and with the treatment team.

For many women with breast cancer, the end of radiation (as in Liz's case) or chemotherapy means the start of taking medication to prevent recurrence. Details about these drugs are presented later in this book, but the concept of recurrence and the fears attached to this concept deserve mention.

All survivors of cancer experience some degree of fear of recurrence. Some people may become hypervigilant and experience panic if they have the odd ache, pain, cough, or sneeze. They may seek medical care more often than necessary and insist on unwarranted tests and investigations. Other survivors attempt to cope by putting the experience behind them by not adhering to after-treatment plans and actively avoiding follow-up care. Neither of these responses is appropriate.

Today, many survivors of cancer are given a survivorship care plan that provides the details of their treatment and recommendations for follow-up care and surveillance. This plan is intended to be shared with the survivor's primary care provider(s) so that appropriate care is provided that is distinct from or a complement to the care provided by the cancer care team.

Chapter 2.
Getting on With Life

January 11, 2010
Start of a great year!

Well, 2010 is here, and I am looking forward to a happy and healthy new year! I finished radiation treatments on December 23 and spent the afternoon celebrating with my sister. It was wonderful.

I made it through the holidays, even though I was extremely exhausted. Every day, I get stronger and have more energy. In fact, I went on my first business trip since the big "C" diagnosis. I have my own consulting business that has suffered a bit since I have been on my cancer journey. I flew to Richmond, Virginia, and worked with a group of board members (Virginia Medical Group Management Association [MGMA], for all of you MGMA folks out there) as the facilitator for their strategic planning retreat. It was great to be out and about and NOT be a patient! I was very tired when I got home (at about 1 am), yet the trip was very gratifying for me professionally.

I have a follow-up visit with the surgeon this Thursday, January 14, and will see the radiation oncologist for a follow-up at the end of the month. My skin is healing and the scar is fading a bit. Not quite ready for the bikini yet!

I am ready to get on with my life and make a difference for others. I'm networking and doing my best to drum up some business so I can work and focus on helping patients—not being one.

Thanks to all of you for your prayers, your cards, your gifts, and (most of all) your support. I am blessed to have such caring people in my life. God bless.

January 2010 to May 18, 2014

All mammograms, scans, and blood work have been fine. I was on tamoxifen for a while until I was postmenopausal. Then, I was on several aromatase inhibitors until the doctor could find one with the least amount of side effects. So many of them caused debilitating joint pain to the point where it was difficult to stand up after a meeting at work. My knees, hips, and other joints were very stiff and painful. I finally ended up on exemestane. I still had joint pain, yet it was tolerable.

Women with hormone receptor-positive breast cancer, often referred to as ER/PR+, are prescribed hormone-blocking medication for a number of years after their primary treatment(s). These medications lower estrogen levels in the blood, preventing the hormone from feeding any cancer cells that still may be in the woman's body, thus reducing the risk of recurrence. Because these medications are given in addition to/after primary treatment, they also are called adjuvant therapies. There are two kinds of medications used for this:

1. Tamoxifen is a SERM and is prescribed to women who are premenopausal to prevent recurrence of cancer. It acts on the breast and vaginal tissues and prevents the body's estrogen from binding with estrogen receptors. It usually is taken for five years.

2. Aromatase inhibitors block the synthesis of estrogen from male hormones (androgens) that are secreted by the adrenal glands. Estrogen is converted from these andro-

gens in the fatty tissues and muscle. Aromatase inhibitors prevent this conversion by acting on enzymes called aromatase enzymes. Aromatase inhibitors are often given to women after they have taken tamoxifen and become postmenopausal. The optimal length of time that these medications should be taken is not clear and is being investigated in clinical trials. Over a 10-year period, aromatase inhibitors may have increased benefit as compared to tamoxifen (Chlebowski et al., 2015).

There are three different types of aromatase inhibitors: exemestane, anastrozole, and letrozole.

Fulvestrant is a selective estrogen receptor downregulator used in postmenopausal women who have experienced disease progression.

All of these medications have side effects that affect quality of life and/or pose a risk to general health.

Tamoxifen is associated with the risk of blood clots and the overgrowth of the lining of the uterus; however, it does prevent osteoporosis and high lipid levels in the blood. It causes hot flashes and vaginal discharge and nausea in some women. The aromatase inhibitors cause joint pain, fatigue, headaches, bone loss with long-term use, hot flashes, and vaginal atrophy. Some women can experience nausea, loss of appetite, insomnia, and anxiety. Weight gain also is reported in women who use these medications. Fulvestrant causes similar symptoms with the addition of cough, shortness of breath, and constipation (Reinbolt et al., 2015).

During this period of time, I attended the Susan G. Komen Race for the Cure every Mother's Day in Pittsburgh and all the Steelers home games during October, at which time I would wear my pink attire. I almost felt a little guilty that I was feeling so great personally yet seeing women who were going through active treatment. On one hand, I felt like my experience was pretty simple. Two lumpectomies and radiation. *Bam.* Done. I didn't need to have any chemotherapy, so I did not go through the same hell that other women have been through. On the other hand, I thought that I should not be so cavalier about my experience and that I was sounding too cocky. That karma always comes back to get you.

Each year before my mammogram, I'd get so incredibly nervous. I would feel great yet would be so scared that the test would reveal something I didn't even feel—just like the one I had in 2009, when I was diagnosed. Dr. G. was the radiologist, and she would always give me the results before I left. She would walk into the waiting area and call me into a changing room. I would intently stare at her face to see if there was any clue as to the results. She then would tell me that everything was fine and hug me. I know, it's a girl thing. I sure looked forward to those hugs! She was so terrific with me and genuinely cared about her patients.

I spent the next four and a half years taking exemestane and living my life. I did some consulting, some traveling to different sites to do presentations, and started a full-time job in April 2011.

Life was good.

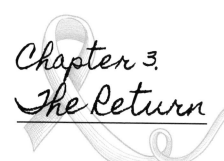

Chapter 3.
The Return

May 19, 2014

My son turned 30 years old today. I can't believe he is that grown up. I worked during the day, and the family all went to dinner together this evening. My dad even joined us. We had a wonderful evening.

May 20, 2014

I woke up in the middle of the night with stabbing right-upper-quadrant abdominal pain that radiated to my right shoulder. I thought it would go away after I got up and got moving. I took a shower, put my big girl clothes on, and went to the local county medical society about 30 minutes from my home.

I spoke at a local conference about health information technology this morning and then stayed for lunch. The pain was increasing. I tried to get an appointment with my primary care provider so as not to abuse those folks in the emergency department (ED), but the gal answering the phone told me to just go to the ED. I did not want to do that but wanted to be seen. At the ED, I was assessed, had a chest x-ray, and had an abdominal CT scan. We waited quite a while before we heard anything.

One of the emergency medicine doctors came in and said they were talking with my oncologist. That really caught me off guard. Why would they be talking to my oncologist? I have abdominal

pain, not anything related to my breasts. He told me he saw something suspicious on my liver but could not be sure. They wanted me
to have an MRI and said that I could get it done as an outpatient. I
left the ED and went home quite puzzled. Again, I never thought
it would be cancer, which was so unusual for me. As a survivor, I
thought every ache and pain was the cancer coming back. I'm not
sure why I didn't think that way this time.

Almost five years after completing primary treatment for
her breast cancer, Liz is experiencing alarming symptoms
suggesting that the cancer may have spread. This is shock-
ing on many levels. For a long time, we thought that if someone was cancer-free after five years, then they were cured. We
now understand that cancer can recur at any time, sometimes
many years later. Like many survivors, Liz worried for a long
time that every symptom, no matter how benign, was a sign
of recurrence. There is evidence that younger women experience greater fear of recurrence (Ziner et al., 2012) in addition to
worries about their general health, their roles as parents and
employees, and fears about losing their "womanhood."

But this time, when Liz experienced severe abdominal
pain, she had no idea that it was caused by the cancer having spread to her liver. In addition, the ED physician was not
completely forthright in talking to her. He first said that he
was talking to Liz's oncologist, which confused her. He then
explained that he had seen something suspicious on the
scan and was not sure what it was. This required further testing—a biopsy of Liz's liver—to confirm his suspicions.

May 22, 2014

Had an MRI as an outpatient.

May 24, 2014

Spoke with my oncologist and reviewed the results of the MRI. Liver has multiple nodules. She could not be sure of anything without a liver biopsy.

May 25 to 27, 2014

Memorial Day weekend. Sat around the pool in lots of pain. Tried to enjoy the pain meds. AGONIZING to wait!

May 28, 2014

Went to my office and met with some of the staff. Gave them a brief update that was very emotional. One of my staff members began to cry. Her sister had just been diagnosed with ovarian cancer a few weeks before this crazy thing happened to me.

May 29, 2014

Had a liver biopsy.

May 30 to June 1, 2014

Going crazy waiting for the results of the biopsy.

Once again, Liz is waiting. It is known that waiting for test results is anxiety provoking. This feeling is worse when the testing performed is invasive and when the patient is new to this kind of testing (Yu, Chojniak, Borba, Girão, & Lourenço, 2011).

June 2, 2014
My diagnosis

Well, I heard the worst possible news today.

Dr. O. said the breast cancer has spread to my entire liver. It is considered stage IV. They still have to run a few more tests to see if this cancer has the same cells as the first one. I am not a candidate for surgery, as my whole liver is affected. I don't know if there is any potential for a liver transplant after the chemotherapy.

Ironically, I had an appointment at the beginning of June with this oncologist that represented my five years of survivorship! Unfortunately, I will not get to celebrate. So sad.

I will see my oncologist on Monday, June 9. We will review the treatment plan. I will need to have full-body scans to see if any other signs of metastasis exist. After that, I will start chemotherapy.

I'm not sure what my schedule will be at this point. I will try to work at least half days, depending on how much pain I am experiencing. Once I know the chemotherapy schedule and how my body will react, I can put together a tentative schedule.

The liver is the third most common site of metastatic spread from a primary breast cancer (bone and lung are more common) and generally suggests a poor prognosis (Charalampoudis et al., 2015). However, some clinicians are using novel approaches to treatment (Schirrmacher, Stücker, Lulei, Bihari, & Sprenger, 2015). Surgical resection to remove malignant lesions is possible in carefully selected patients.

After the phone call, I was absolutely hysterical. Stage IV is a death sentence! I still have so much to live for, especially when it comes to my children. They already are living without one parent. I cannot abandon them! I want to see them finish college, get married, and have babies. I want to be a grandma!

I just lay on my bed sobbing. No one was around. I texted my husband and asked him to come right home. His office was about 10 minutes away, and he came home and heard me crying. I kept telling him that I was going to die and that I did not want to die yet. He tried to comfort me as best as he could. He finally got me settled down enough for me to explain what had happened. At this point, I did not know that stage IV meant that the original cancer had metastasized to another place. I just thought it was the end. These were the most awful feelings of my life. It was very painful when my daughter died and painful when my second husband died. However, thinking about my own mortality and the children I would leave behind was more than I could handle. I felt like I was having a mental breakdown.

The most common fear for women with breast cancer is fear of recurrence. For Liz, the recurrence is in the form of metastasis (or distant spread) of the cancer to her liver. The recommended treatment for this is chemotherapy, as the disease is regarded as having systemic spread in this instance (Seidensticker et al., 2015).

Cancer, despite increasingly positive outcomes for those diagnosed with early-stage cancer, still is a threat to life. Liz's reaction to this new diagnosis reflects this existential threat and clearly conveys that cancer also is a threat to one's identity (Leveälahti, Tishelman, & Öhlén, 2007)—in Liz's case, her identity as a mother and future grandmother.

After my kids' father died, I kept telling them how Dad was alive one minute and dead the next. He died at the top of his game. He had been promoted to vice president for the company he worked for and was really happy. At least we did not have to watch him suffer with something such as cancer.

When I was diagnosed with cancer in 2009, I waited awhile to tell them. I can't believe I had used that scenario when talking about their dad, and here I was being diagnosed with cancer. I just never thought it would happen to me. They actually took it very well because I didn't look sick. They weren't at the hospital for the surgery, they didn't see me going to radiation treatments, and I didn't complain about things in front of them. Ashley W. thought I didn't have cancer anymore because it was cut out during the surgery.

When it came back in 2014 and they realized I would have to have chemotherapy, they were worried. Ashley W. saw something with stage IV on it and knew that was very bad. She came to me crying and said she couldn't live without me. She said that she did not want to be an orphan. Her words cut right through my heart. I tried to comfort her as much as I could. I told her I was doing everything the doctors and nurses wanted me to do. I also thought that she might feel better being involved in my care, although not when I was really sick from the chemotherapy.

In particular, women with cancer often feel the need to support distressed family members. In some ways, this allows them to play their usual role as mother and protector. In other ways, it deprives them of the support they may need. A study from the United Kingdom suggests that some survivors of cancer play their usual roles and keep their precancer routines and identity in order to minimize the effect the cancer has on their lives (Baker et al., 2014). In Liz's case, her husband is her primary support and she has to rethink the way she has protected her daughter in the past. Now, Liz needs to involve Ashley W. and keep her informed about what is going on. Gradually informing family about bad news was shown to be the preferred method of communication in one study (Deschepper et al., 2008). For many survivors of cancer, the additional stress the diagnosis places on family is a primary concern (Kutner, Steiner, Corbett, Jahnigen, & Barton, 1999).

June 9, 2014

Just got home from an oncologist visit. For those of you who understand all this stuff, I am ER+ (just like the first time). They will know tomorrow about my HER2/neu status.

If it is negative (like last time), I will start capecitabine this week. It is an oral chemotherapy drug that I will take two times per day for 14 days. I then will have seven days off before restarting the cycle. No hair loss here. I think the oncologist was basing this treatment on the fact that I did not want to lose my hair. However, I certainly don't want to lose my life.

If it is positive, I will receive the following IV infusions every three weeks, starting this week: docetaxel, trastuzumab, and pertuzumab. I will have the first dose peripherally and then get a port inserted for ongoing treatments. My hair will fall out approximately 14–21 days after the start of the docetaxel.

Chemotherapy, either intravenously or in pill form, is prescribed based on a number of factors, including whether the tumor has estrogen, progesterone, or HER2/neu receptors. Over the years, research has attempted to establish the most effective medications and the best ways of using these medications to maximize effectiveness and minimize harm to the patient. Chemotherapy attacks rapidly dividing cells, including cancer and other tissues in the body that divide rapidly, such as hair and mucous membranes (in the mouth and genital areas). This causes side effects that can make life very difficult.

I will get a full-body positron-emission tomography (PET) scan soon, if the insurance approves it. If not, they will do CTs instead.

I specifically asked Dr. O. about a time frame. I had to push hard to get her to give me an idea. She said maybe two years . . . I told her, "I have kids," and "I can't leave them!" It was terrifying to hear her words. I know I pushed her and was happy to have some idea of what she was thinking. However, I will do everything I can to live beyond two years.

That's all for now. More to follow tomorrow.

Giving bad news is challenging, even for experienced healthcare providers. It requires great skill and caring to communicate with patients and avoid unnecessary distress and hopelessness. When healthcare providers deliver a poor prognosis using a positive frame ("You have a 30% chance of surviving") rather than a negative frame ("You have a 70% chance of dying"), patients are more hopeful and less distressed (Porensky & Carpenter, 2015). Patients have been shown to perceive a physician as more compassionate when they give a message with more optimism than a physician who gives the same message with a less optimistic message (Tanco et al., 2015).

Patients given a positively framed message also were more likely to recall the information they were given accurately. It is important that patients are given accurate information about their prognosis so that they can plan for the life they have left. This especially is important for those who have children and have recently received a diagnosis (Umezawa, Fujimori, Matsushima, Kinoshita, & Uchitomi, 2015).

However, predicting survival is difficult and usually inaccurate. In one study, survival time was overestimated 26% of the time and underestimated 28% of the time (Taniyama et al., 2014). Overestimating survival may lead to patients not being able to prepare for their shortened life span and may result in plans for end-of-life care to being neglected if patients think that they have more time left than they really do.

June 10, 2014

Talked to my oncology nurse today. My HER2/neu status is negative, so I will start on oral capecitabine as soon as we fight with the insurance company to get it approved. The office is completing the documentation, and then I will get a call from the pharmacy. My nurse, Karen, told me that if the pharmacy calls and says the co-pay will be $2,000 per month, don't give them my credit card. They will work with the cancer center case manager to get a more realistic co-pay. Thank goodness.

The office also is sending the paperwork through to the insurer to get the full-body PET scan covered. If insurance says no, they will do a bone scan and then individual CT scans of the rest of my body.

Right now, I am trying to work about four hours per day, usually in the afternoon or early evening, as I am so tired in the morning. I'll keep you posted.

P.S. Trying hard to keep my sense of humor . . .

Humor can be an effective way to cope with difficult situations. Positive humor (humor that is self-effacing or affiliative) is thought to enhance mental toughness, which also is thought to encourage humor (Veselka, Schermer, Martin, & Vernon, 2010). In the context of cancer care, humor can be used as a coping mechanism and also enhances the relationship between patient and nurse. Trust needs to be established first in order for the expression of humor, especially if it is initiated by the nurse, to be acceptable to the patient (Tanay, Roberts, & Ream, 2013). Humor is thought to alleviate anxiety, and many patients appreciate humor from their healthcare providers (Rose, Spencer, & Rausch, 2013). Patients who use humor to cope with their illness are seen as emotionally healthy. This applies when the humor is directed toward the cancer experience itself and not just as a general attitude (Shapiro, McCue, Heyman, Dey, & Haller, 2010).

June 11, 2014

Today would have been Amanda's 27th birthday. R.I.P. my Amanda Panda.

I spent some time talking with friends and colleagues. The nurses at the Oncology Nursing Society (ONS) were amazing. They shared some of their knowledge with me, as did some other people. I decided to seek a second opinion. I just didn't feel that Dr. O. was being aggressive enough, especially after she gave me only two years. I want an aggressive treatment to give me the best chance at life.

June 12, 2014

I am scheduled to see another oncologist (Dr. L.) on June 18 to get a second opinion. He is with the same organization as the first doctor. He also is affiliated with a nationally known National Cancer Institute–designated comprehensive cancer center. He is the chief of their breast cancer program. He will have access to all of my scans and blood work because their system is all connected electronically. (This is one of the reasons I chose them during my first round with breast cancer—hoping it keeps medical errors to a minimum!)

It is not unusual for patients to seek a second opinion on various aspects of their care—from the diagnosis itself to management. A review of studies on second opinions suggests that 10%–62% of second opinions result in a significant change in the diagnosis, treatment plan, or prognosis. Patients tend to request a second opinion when they are dissatisfied with the original consultation with a physician, if they want additional information, or if they experience persistent symptoms or complications from treatment (Payne et al., 2014). A second opinion may be requested even when there are clear guidelines for the management of a particular condition (Moumjid, Gafni, Bremond, & Carrere, 2007). A second opinion also may result in investigations being repeated at both a financial cost and risk to patient health; however, the patient may feel this is worthwhile. One study resulted in 70% of patients receiving beneficial advice (Mustafa, Bijl, & Gans, 2002). Not all physicians welcome a patient seeking a second opinion and may feel offended, resentful, and embarrassed (Greenfield, Pliskin, Feder-Bubis, Wientroub, & Davidovitch, 2012). In oncology, patients who are female, younger, and more educated appear to seek a second opinion more often in order to receive additional information about their treatment plan or reassurance that the plan is appropriate (Tattersall et al., 2009).

This afternoon, my work peeps came to my house for our regular monthly meeting (instead of meeting at the office). It was so wonderful to see all of them and we had a productive meeting. They all have been so incredibly supportive.

Social support is universally regarded as an important part of coping with breast and other cancers. Support from friends was stated as the second most frequent source (after family) in a study of women with breast cancer (Raupach & Hiller, 2002). Women who have supportive social networks have better outcomes after breast cancer; even small social networks that provide high support serve to create better outcomes. The quality of the support is what counts (Kroenke et al., 2013). Social support is noted to increase post-traumatic growth (the positive personal growth that many people report after going through a traumatic experience), and a combination of supportive friends who provide information to the woman with breast cancer is important (Hasson-Ohayon et al., 2015).

So, I still am playing the waiting game. The pain is not as intense, so I have cut back on the pain meds. I usually can get through the day and then take one in the early evening and one before I go to bed.

June 18, 2014
Second opinion

I went to the cancer center today for a second opinion. I met with two physicians—one was an oncology fellow and one was a well-known oncologist. The meeting was great, and it is the first time in the last month that I have had some hope.

I am having a full-body PET scan tomorrow at the hospital and having a venous port inserted on Friday, June 20. The new plan is to start docetaxel (IV chemotherapy, which will cause hair loss) and capecitabine (oral chemotherapy and no hair loss) on Tuesday of next week. This plan is more aggressive in order to get the cancer under control a bit faster. The doctor also gave me some new pain meds in the hopes of getting my pain under control.

I will be getting more information from several folks tomorrow. I just got home, am in pain, and am quite tired. I'll post more tomorrow.

P.S. For those of you at work, I still am trying to come in to the office on Monday, June 23, for our division's event. I can show off my new port!

June 26, 2014
Chemotherapy has started

I had the port implanted on Monday. All went well. It is quite sore and tender, but I am told the soreness will improve with time.

A port is a device that is implanted under the skin on the upper chest through which chemotherapy and other IV therapies can be administered. It is used instead of a peripheral IV line inserted into a superficial vein in the arm for a number of reasons. These include a decrease in the risk of infection, protection of the patient's veins from chemotherapy that causes pain or damages veins, and better quality of life for patients, as they can carry on their usual activities without concern that they will harm themselves or the tubing and needle in the arm. Other advantages include the ability of nurses to access the device much quicker than a traditional IV and the fact that the patient's skin protects the device (Kreis et al., 2007). But, as Liz experienced, it can hurt the first few times that the port is accessed, as a needle has to puncture the skin. These devices generally are very safe and stay in the patient's body until the end of treatment (Ignatov et al., 2009).

I had my first IV treatment with docetaxel on Tuesday. Yes, I made sure it was Pink Tuesday, just like every Tuesday at work. However, this time it had a lot more meaning. Whew. It really hurt when the nurse accessed the port. I yelled, "Ouch!" and scared the guy next to me! After that, it was business as usual.

The oncology nurses were fabulous! They all were ONS members, and some of them had their certification. It was great to see ONS in action through these dedicated folks.

The actual chemotherapy infusion only took about an hour. They gave me several IV meds before the docetaxel to help with the side effects. We were home around 1 pm.

Today, it is standard practice to give medications before starting IV chemotherapy to reduce the risk of acute reactions, such as nausea and vomiting. These medications are commonly called "supportive care agents" and are prescribed depending on the side effects of each specific chemotherapy agent that is given to the patient.

It's kind of weird. Today is day 3, and I am waiting for these awful side effects to hit me. So far, I feel pretty good (knock on wood). I certainly don't want to jinx myself.

I also started the capecitabine (another chemotherapy drug) by mouth last night. I took my second dose today and already have been using the cream on my hands and feet to prevent dryness.

Capecitabine is an oral (taken by mouth) treatment for cancer (Saif, Katirtzoglou, & Syrigos, 2008). The drug is broken down into a potent anticancer agent within the cancer cells and, because of this, has fewer toxic side effects, particularly on the bone marrow. Because this is given in pill form and taken by the patient at home, education about potential side effects is important. It also is extremely important that the patient understands when to take the medication, how to store it safely, and why it is important to take it at the prescribed time. If a dose is missed, the patient should not double up on the next dose. It also is important not to take the medication during the "off week."

Side effects of capecitabine include hand-foot syndrome, which ranges from numbness, tingling, redness, and/or discomfort in the hands and feet (grade 1); to redness and swelling that is painful (grade 2); to skin breakdown, ulcers, and severe pain that interferes with the patient's ability to walk or do their usual daily activities (grade 3). Other side effects include diarrhea, mouth ulcers, nausea and vomiting, abdominal pain, and loss of appetite. Damage to the heart (cardiotoxicity) is a rare but severe side effect of the drug.

I am quite tired yet feel guilty just lying on the couch watching TV. However, I am learning that resting is the best thing I could be doing right now.

Darcie, my friend and amazing hairdresser, cut my hair really short last night. It is a stepping stone. It feels really weird yet is so much cooler! We are going to visit the wig place on Monday, June 30, to pick out some sassy hairstyles for when my hair falls out, which should be in about two weeks.

Preparing for the eventual hair loss associated with chemotherapy is one way of coping with this side effect, viewed as one of the worst by women. Depending on the specific chemotherapy, hair loss in women may be total or they may experience thinning. Everyone experiences this loss differently. Liz's decision to cut her hair short is, as she says, a "stepping stone" to acclimate to what comes next.

My husband has been absolutely amazing. Boy, I sure love that man. He has been so helpful during my little pity parties and is the best support I could ever ask for. Ashley E. also has been wonderful cleaning the house and making me some lime Jell-O—my favorite. She has spent much more time at home.

I get cards every day in the mail, which I so appreciate. I LOVE cards, and I'm like a little kid when the mail gets here.

Thank you to everyone. I so enjoy hearing from you, your kind words, and your faith in me to beat this thing. I have been focusing on the negatives, and you all are helping me to be more positive and to focus on healing and survivorship. You have no idea how this support is helping me.

That's all for now. I hear the couch calling my name.

Family is the most important source of support for women with breast cancer (Kolokotroni, Anagnostopoulos, & Tsikkinis, 2014). A partner who is supportive and caring provides a safe space for women where they can assimilate the distress they are experiencing and find ways to turn that into post-traumatic growth (Weiss, 2004).

June 30, 2014

Today, I felt like hell; so dehydrated. Spent all afternoon at the cancer center, where they drained a liter of fluid from my abdomen. (That's 1,000 cc or ml for those of you still challenged by the metric system.) Went home and struggled through the rest of the day. Tomorrow also would have been my mom's 82nd birthday—the second birthday since she died. Sad day.

July 1, 2014

Woke up with chills and leg cramps and a feeling like I was going to die. Went to the cancer center around 9 am, spent all day there, and was admitted to the hospital that night. I had neutropenic fever, severe dehydration, severe mucositis, and needed serious pain management.

Febrile neutropenia is a common side effect of chemotherapy and refers to a high temperature due to low white cell counts. White blood cells (WBCs) are part of the body's immune system, and their role is to fight infection. As has been explained previously, chemotherapy attacks rapidly dividing cells, and WBCs fall into this category. When white cell counts are low, patients are at risk of acquired (new) infections and also reactivation of latent infections in the body that have been prevented by a healthy immune system (Virizuela et al., 2016).

This is regarded as an emergency, and treatment should be given promptly, usually with IV antibiotics. Patients with febrile neutropenia usually are very sick and feel terrible. They often are admitted to a hospital not only for antibiotic treatment, but also because they may need other supportive medication, oxygen, and intensive nursing and medical care. In order to reduce further complications, some EDs have special protocols for patients with cancer who present with febrile neutropenia, allowing antibiotic treatment within a much shorter time frame of 90 minutes (Keng et al., 2015).

NOTE TO ALL: I have been on a patient-controlled analgesia (PCA) with hydromorphone to manage my pain, so there may be misspelled words or improper English.

Pain is an expected and much-feared symptom of cancer and cancer treatments. PCA allows the patient to control the frequency of small amounts of pain medication through an IV. Each time the patient pushes a button on a handheld device, a small, preprogrammed amount of pain medication is infused. This method of pain control has been used for many years in patients after surgery, but its use in controlling cancer pain is fairly new. It has been shown to be safe in this population (Sousa et al., 2014).

I won't go through every detail about this admission because IT AIN'T PRETTY! My husband, who has no medical background, has learned more things about my body than I think I even knew.

To be honest, I was afraid I was going to die. I mean that very seriously. I wanted them to keep me alive until Ashley W. got home from her semester abroad in Europe. My other two kids were in college no more than 90 minutes away, so they could make it home rather quickly. I had just seen my other family members over the weekend. It was the most frightening event of my life. I think you get the point.

Anyhow, the doctors and especially the nurses miraculously raised me from the dead. I am still here. I'll give you more details when some of these drugs wear off. My counts are coming back up, so I am starting to feel a bit better. I hope to be home early next week.

The one thing that was most important to me was patient safety. I finished my dissertation in June 2013 and received my PhD in August of that year. I had been researching patient safety, medical errors, and health information technology for five years! I was very nervous about becoming the victim of an error. Therefore, from the start, I asked the nurses about what they were giving me. I would ask the name of the medication, the dosage, what it did, etc. I even asked the nursing aide/patient care technician for my vitals and temperature, which I wrote down every time they took them. Some of them realized how important that need was for me and turned the machine around so I could see it and write down the numbers. A few of them were a bit put off, yet they complied with my request.

A medical or nursing error is a source of great distress for patients—made worse if they are not told why an error occurred. The most common errors involve medication (wrong drug, dose, patient, time, or route). Communication errors and those related to coordination of care are the next most common experienced by patients (Harrison et al., 2015). Nurses have to take a number of precautions in order to provide safe care when giving medications to patients. These include the safe preparation and administration of medication, understanding the risks inherent in administering medications and knowing how to do this safely to protect from errors, and being aware of how work pressure can lead to errors. However, it is not just a matter of following protocols that helps to prevent errors; clinical judgment and reasoning about patients and their condition is an important part of keeping them safe and avoiding errors (Smeulers, Onderwater, van Zwieten, & Vermeulen, 2014). This means that sometimes a nurse might withhold medication, even though it has been prescribed for a patient, because taking it may make the patient's condition worse. Using clinical judgment, nurses would contact the healthcare provider who prescribed the medication and report their findings and ask for a change of medication. The use of information technology has helped to avoid medication errors (Choo, Hutchinson, & Bucknall, 2010); computer programs remove the risk of transcription errors (physician prescriptions that are not legible), and dispensing systems reduce the risk that the wrong dose of a medication will be given. In addition, using bar code scanners to check that the right patient receives the correct medication is another safety initiative designed to reduce medication errors.

July 4, 2014
To hell and back

Well, I have been a patient in the hospital since Wednesday, July 2. I have never been an inpatient during July 4th festivities. No fireworks for me.

July 6, 2014
Update

Keep the cards coming. They are so inspirational to me. I love them.

We have lots of plants and flowers, so save your money there. ☺

My husband always offers to cut my hair for me and save us some money. I have always said to him, "No, thank you." Well, today was his chance. He brought the kitchen shears from home (don't worry, they were clean) at my request. My scalp is itchy and sore, so I asked him to chop away. I will be posting some pics some time when I have more energy. He did a great job, and the back of my head feels so much better.

I'm getting my head shaved tomorrow. Darcie is coming to the hospital with all of her "stuff." My sister will be here, too. Some pretty scarves would be much appreciated.

Some patients decide to shave their head, either in anticipation of losing all their hair or because they hate it falling out bit by bit and finding chunks of hair in their bed, on their pillows, in the shower, and on furniture. No matter the motivation to do this, it is a challenge, as many women like their hair, and being bald has a significant influence on body image and how women view themselves when they look in the mirror.

In one study, 55% of women experienced distress from losing their hair; this was associated with poorer body image, psychosocial well-being, and overall health (Choi et al., 2014). It is important to remember that for some women, hair loss means loss of ALL hair on the body, including pubic hair, eyelashes, eyebrows, and other body hair. Not having hair is a visible sign to the world that you have cancer, and this can be very distressing (Roe, 2011).

There is not much that can be done about chemotherapy-associated hair loss on the head. Scalp cooling has shown some benefits (Shin, Jo, Kim do, Kwon, & Myung, 2015), but it is expensive, has to be used with each chemotherapy session, and is not always available at cancer centers. Concerns also have been raised about the risk of cancer on the scalp if chemotherapy does not reach the hair follicles that are cooled. However, these concerns seem to be in patients with blood cancers rather than with breast and other solid cancers.

I will let you know when I can eat again.

I also love lilac candles.

I am continuing to make clinical progress. Cardiac monitor is off. One major antibiotic was discontinued. Two other IV meds were finished. I won't be going home until multiple issues are addressed (eating, drinking, pain control, etc.), yet I am making good progress.

I continue to thank God for the ability to keep recovering. I am blessed to have all of you in my life and ask for your continued prayers. I draw strength from you.

Hugs and love to all of my prayer warriors. ♥

July 7, 2014
Still in the hospital

Lots of milestones reached today.

Saw my regular oncologist after three days over the big holiday weekend. Caught up on everything.

Several meds were discontinued, which to me says one step closer to out the door! Walked several laps around the unit. Felt great to exercise my legs. My husband was my official escort. Felt like we were going to the prom.

Darcie came over and buzzed my hair. There still are some nubs left that might fall out in a week or so. Tony, her hubby and a survivor of cancer, was her chauffeur to this part of town. Everyone said my head looked cute bald, as it was nice and round. However, I looked in the mirror and cried. Now, I look like a frail patient with cancer. I am so sad.

Patty was here for the afternoon, serving as the official photographer for the hair event. She did a great job. In all seriousness, I don't know what I would do without my beautiful sister.

I had laser work on the lesions in my mouth (mucositis); a bit too yucky for those of you nonmedical folks. I will have it once per day for the next few days to help the ulcers heal. I did some research via my peeps to get more details about this laser treatment. Many of them talked with my doctor after I had already introduced the idea. He originally said no. He came in and said to me, "And don't think you can send your friends to me to change my mind!" I was so impressed that he knew I was well connected. He eventually caved in after I suggested a compromise. I felt so good! I still have some influence over what is happening to me.

And then . . . I had my first taste of real food in weeks. Mashed potatoes. Tasted like filet mignon! Again, one more positive step in my chemotherapy cycle 1 recovery.

Mucositis is caused by inflammation and breakdown of the inner lining of the mouth, throat, and esophagus. Mucous membranes are composed of rapidly dividing cells; chemotherapy attacks these cells, causing breakdown and ulcers. This is extremely painful and the person often cannot eat or drink, take oral medications for pain, swallow, brush their teeth, or even talk.

When a patient develops mucositis, it may be necessary to reduce the dose of chemotherapy or stop treatment for a while to allow healing to occur. Ulcers in the mouth increase the risk of developing an infection, especially in a patient who has a compromised immune system from chemotherapy. Weight loss is common if a patient cannot eat or drink, and some patients require IV feeding to maintain their nutritional status (Al-Ansari et al., 2015).

Few effective treatments exist for oral mucositis. Prevention using ice (cryotherapy) has been suggested and was shown to be effective in patients receiving 5-fluorouracil. Other suggested treatments include good mouth care; drugs such as palifermin, allopurinol, and chlorhexidine; and supplements such as zinc sulfate; these require further study before becoming part of routine treatment (Manzi, Silveira, & Reis, 2016). Many of these studies have been done in the context of radiation-induced mucositis, and results may not be transferable to chemotherapy-induced mucositis (Van Sebille et al., 2015). Little evidence exists supporting natural remedies, such as honey, aloe vera, or essential oils (Agham-ohamamdi & Hosseinimehr, 2016).

Low-level laser therapy has been suggested for both the prevention and treatment of mucositis. A review of this modality concluded that while positive results have been seen in patients with chemotherapy-induced mucositis, not enough evidence exists to recommend its use at this time (Migliorati et al., 2013).

When I was working at another hospital/level I trauma center in this area, we used to train the new residents before they started on July 1 of each year. We used to joke around that you never want to be in the hospital when the residents start on July 1. Well, I was in the hospital to mark that milestone. In fact, I kind of befriended one of the residents. It was clear that he was clueless to the whole oncology thing. I tried to teach HIM a few things, and it made me feel good to be using my nursing skills for someone else. I also learned that I could recommend changes in my treatment that he then would take to the physician. These changes were strongly considered coming from the physician instead of the patient. See, I am still working the system.

I have officially decided to write a book and am keeping lots of notes. Early this am (5 to be exact), I took a bunch of pictures of my IV "tree" (as my friend called it), my list of meds, the computer screens, etc.

So, I am celebrating the small successes. Let's see what tomorrow brings.

July 10, 2014
Progress continues!

Yesterday marked one week since I have been in the hospital. It feels like I have been here for at least two weeks. In the beginning, each day felt like three days—morning, evening, and night shifts. I was so sick and in so much pain that each shift felt like another day. However, like Kiefer Sutherland says in the show *24*, I was determined to "live another day!" I somehow got through each set of 24 hours . . . one hour at a time.

> Being in a hospital is difficult for most people and especially difficult for nurses! Time takes on a different meaning when one is sick and in pain; it often feels like it is going backward. Liz describes this so well when she says that each eight-hour shift felt like a day to her; pain alters one's perception of time.

OK, on to more positive things. I am able to see the progress I have made and am regaining control of my own health. This concept is incredibly important, as it serves as a type of self-motivator. It is helping me to heal, as that helpless feeling SUCKED and served as a major reason for my despair and ongoing discouragement.

> Being diagnosed with a recurrence of cancer is in many ways worse than an initial diagnosis. The shock of the first diagnosis is tempered over time by treatment and the hope and expectation of cure. When the cancer recurs, hope often is lost at least temporarily, and for some women, the realization that their life is likely to be shorter than expected can lead to feelings of hopelessness and despair (Warren, 2009).
>
> Poor quality of sleep, depression, and fatigue contribute to the experience of distress (Mosher & DuHamel, 2012). Being in the hospital usually means poor sleep because of unfamiliar surroundings; multiple disturbances during the night from noise, lights, and other patients; and interruptions for nursing care.

Patient satisfaction is an important factor in hospitals today. Patients frequently are asked to evaluate their experiences. Inconveniences and errors may cause dissatisfaction, and women with breast cancer have been found to be clear on what they will excuse and what they won't. Davoll et al. (2013) found that 48% of the women they surveyed were prepared to overlook small disruptions while in the hospital, a third were prepared to accept lack of cleanliness and other "unfavorable" conditions, and 53.6% were willing to excuse service that they regarded as less than desirable. These patients were willing to accept less than desirable service because they thought that staff was busy and had high demands placed on them. This study suggests that many hospitalized women make excuses for poor service and accept what they are provided with, resulting in feelings of dissatisfaction with their care.

I am continuing to reintroduce foods. Can't wait for my hospital cinnamon oatmeal for breakfast. I may even try some tea with cream. Don't worry, I also have protein coming—a scrambled egg. Hey, I'm going all out here.

The PCA pump was removed yesterday. This change was a HUGE step in my healing. It was so easy to push the button when I felt pain, which at times was very severe. Between liquid pain meds and advancing my diet to food that I could tolerate, I was OK going the oral route.

The other antibiotics and the peripheral IV in my left arm also were removed. I see each of these actions as one more tile on the floor building me a path to go home.

Last (but most important of the entire day), one of the pastors from my church stopped by to visit me. He has a small church about 90 minutes from Pittsburgh. He drove all the way down here to see me. OK, maybe that is a bit of an exaggeration. He had been in the Pittsburgh area for other things. We had a great visit, and he prayed with me and my husband. Did I cry? Of course.

Have to get ready for my gourmet breakfast.

Pssst . . . I might get to go home today. Don't want to say it too loud and jinx things.

Religious faith and practice have been shown to have positive effects on various aspects of quality of life, including a sense of meaning and peace for people with advanced cancer (Bai, Lazenby, Jeon, Dixon, & McCorkle, 2015). Researchers have found that those who have strong faith experience less anxiety and depression (Johnson et al., 2011) and have improved functional quality of life (Canada, Murphy, Fitchett, & Stein, 2016). Praying has been shown to improve body acceptance in women with breast cancer (Paiva et al., 2013). Survivors of breast cancer with a strong faith practice may focus on self-improvement or helping others as a way of incorporating their faith in everyday life (Schreiber & Edward, 2015).

July 10, 2014
Update

HOME!!!
HOME!
HOME!
HOME!
HOME!
HOME!
HOME!
Get it? Exhausted. More tomorrow.

July 11, 2014
The journey home

Well, I made it home! What a fabulous feeling to step out of the hospital (OK, be rolled out in a wheelchair) and feel the sun on my face, smell the grass, and feel the breeze across my face. We take so many things for granted in this life, and these simple smells and feelings are so appreciated when they have been taken away—even for just a week.

Being the expert planner I am, I thought my strategy was going well. I had taken my regular meds, my antinausea med, and, most importantly, my pain med to make sure I had good coverage until I got home and could take the next dose.

We got to our neighborhood grocery store/pharmacy and went in the drive-through lane. My husband handed the girl my prescriptions. I heard, "We don't have that one. It's not very common." She was talking about the pain medication. I suggested that they give me 10 cc and then order the remaining amount. She talked to the pharmacist, who said they didn't have it. Period. No other suggestions. Shitty customer service per my compromised state.

"Sucks for you to be in pain. Next customer?"

Of course, I plan to send a letter to the president of the chain to express my sincere disappointment, make some recommendations, and offer to present a customer service program for the pharmacy staff.

We went to two other pharmacies with no luck. The staff at the second pharmacy was much friendlier and gave us some other suggestions. I told my husband we should have had it filled at the hospital before we left, yet I never thought of that idea. I was disappointed that someone from my care team did not double-check on the availability of this much of a pain drug.

A successful hospital stay is based not only on the patient recovering from the illness or emergency that precipitated the admission, but also on how the patient is prepared for discharge. The patient needs verbal and written instructions on what to expect when they are home, what symptoms to look for that indicate a need to seek further care, and clear instructions about when to see their primary care provider or specialist for postdischarge follow-up.

Liz's description of going home without pain medication or access to the medication that she needs is an example of how things can go wrong. Not having adequate pain control quite easily can become a reason for a visit to an ED and/or readmission to the hospital. That would be emotionally and financially expensive for Liz and her family.

We got home. I was exhausted—mentally and physically—as well as in significant pain. I lay down on my bed while my husband was on the phone with the oncologist's nurse navigator and other folks at the hospital. The hospital pharmacy was making arrangements to fill the prescription for the pain medicine. However, we would have to drive down to the hospital and back—about a two-hour round trip with traffic. It was the only way we could get the drug tonight.

I woke up in a panic, not knowing where I was or what was happening. I began to cry, and all of the frustration and fright and pain came pouring out. My husband already had worked out the details and did his best to comfort me.

No matter how much planning I had done, I could not replicate the efficiency or safety of the hospital. Again, I was at the mercy of others who knew nothing about me. I had no control over my own health, pain control, etc. It was unbelievably discouraging.

Being discharged from the hospital and having the sense of loss of safety from being observed and cared for is a frequent experience for patients. It is frightening, stressful, and (especially for Liz) discouraging.

People need different things when they come home after being in the hospital. For some, it is written instructions about when to take medications or when to follow up with their primary care provider, oncologist, rehabilitation specialist, etc. Others need more support in terms of emotional care. A Danish study (Mikkelsen, Sondergaard, Jensen, & Olesen, 2008) reports that recently discharged patients wanted five major issues addressed:

1. Support and information on rehabilitation
2. Support for their family members
3. Psychological support to address their fear of the cancer coming back
4. Social support needs
5. Understanding how their friends and family might relate to them

Even though Liz is a nurse, she is first and foremost a patient. Despite her knowledge and experience as a nurse, going home after an intensive level of nursing and medical care was a frightening experience.

My sister works at a college close to the hospital where I was discharged. My husband talked with her, and she will pick up the bottle of pain medicine. Patty and Ashley E. then will meet halfway between the hospital and our home to "make the exchange." Sounds like a drug deal, doesn't it? I just cannot believe that no one even gave us the heads up. Poor care coordination, in my opinion. We could have gotten the script filled at the hospital, saving me a lot of fear and apprehension. I already was a bit nervous about going home, as I won't have someone watching over me and delivering meds in a controlled atmosphere. My husband has been great as my caregiver, but there is only so much he can do. Geez!

Tomorrow: Better days ahead.

July 11, 2014
First full day at home

After all the craziness of yesterday, today was a much better day. I am on what my husband calls "hospital time." Anyone who has been in the hospital or has taken care of patients knows that something's always happening when you are really sick. I was used to being awake every hour or every two hours as I started to get better—blood draws for lab work, vital signs, machines beeping as medications were finished, more meds to hang, etc. The nurses did their best not to wake me, yet I was way too nosey and wanted to know everything that was being done.

I am someone that likes to sleep in on the weekend when I don't have to get up for work. Sleeping until 11 am is not unusual for me. Today, I was wide awake at 6 am and had *Good Morning America* on by 7 am. Finally, by 7:30 am, I asked my husband, "What time is breakfast served around these parts?" Hint, hint, hint. I was used to eating small amounts of food frequently, so I was hungry.

He did a great job feeding me and making sure I had whatever I needed. I keep saying this. I could not get through this treatment without his loving support. Thank you, Lord, for giving me such a loving partner.

The other exciting part about this day is that Ashley W. flew home from Europe! She landed in Philadelphia around 5 pm. She called me first from her friend's phone. It was so great to hear her voice! She was standing in a long line at customs to get back into the

United States. Luckily, they let her back in. Ha ha! Her boyfriend picked her up, and they'll be staying at his house tonight.

Overall, a good day.

July 11 to 12, 2014
Adjusting to my new home schedule

Each day gets better, as I am adjusting to my new schedule at home. I still wake up every hour or two and try hard to roll over and go back to sleep. Some nights are easier than others. I usually am up between 6 and 7 am and now can make my own tea and breakfast without having to depend on anyone. Hello, independence! I have missed you!

I have been active during the day. To my work peeps: You would be so proud of me. I am the poster child of Get Up, Get Moving to decrease my fatigue and increase my stamina. I started off going around the dining room table. I then graduated to walking around the pool a few times then to walking the perimeter of the house. I am a slow mover yet am getting stronger each day. I have my earphones on, I'm listening to music, and I am singing my heart out as I walk. I look and sound a bit silly, although my hubby is happy to see me happy and moving around. He still makes fun of me to keep my sense of humor intact. I love that guy. It is difficult to walk on the grass, so I need more practice to get my muscles back in shape. Lying in bed will do that to you.

Physical activity is a vital part of recovery from cancer treatment. In many ways, Liz indeed is the poster child. The American Cancer Society/American Society of Clinical Oncology Breast Cancer Survivorship Care Guideline (Runowicz et al., 2016) recommends 150 minutes of moderate exercise weekly or 75 minutes of vigorous exercise each week. Strength training should be included twice a week, particularly for women on endocrine therapy or chemotherapy.

Exercise is known to have several benefits for survivors of breast cancer during and after treatment, including promoting psychological and physical wellness, providing a distraction from being ill, and feeling supported by family and friends who join them in their exercise efforts (Husebø, Allan, Karlsen, Søreide, & Bru, 2015). Physical activity also has been shown to reduce the risk of death from breast cancer (Lahart, Metsios, Nevill, & Carmichael, 2015).

July 13, 2014

I was up early before anyone (as usual) and took some time to do my hair. Psych! It took about 10 seconds to dry off my head. Wow, this buzz cut is such a time saver. I ate breakfast, put on some clean clothes, and went to church! My son's friend Justin drove me, dropped me off, and came back for me at 11 am. The hour at church was so powerful for me. Our usual pastor is on a sabbatical for the summer, so we had another person covering whom I had never met. I still felt him talking to me, especially since there weren't too many people there. I cried through half of the service because I was so grateful that God had carried me through this first cycle of treatment. I was able to take communion, which helped strengthen me and carried the grace of God through my body. More grateful tears. I left feeling renewed and ready to go through cycle 2 on Tuesday. I plan to go each week as I am able and as my counts are good.

Justin was my personal chauffeur for the day! We went to Patrick's softball game for a bit. Justin set up my chair, got out the umbrella to keep me out of the sun, and helped with anything I wanted. I really like this service!

We left there and went to pick up Ashley W. She was able to come home from State College, Pennsylvania, with one of her roommates from last year. This gal lives in the town where I grew up, which is about 30 minutes from our house! We pulled up to the house, and I saw Ashley standing on the front step. I immediately started to cry (and have serious tears in my eyes as I write this update) and thanked God for her safe return to us. Patrick was with us and was very happy to see his baby sister. She came over to the car, I hugged her, and we both cried. I felt like I did not want to let her go. When she left for Europe, I had all of my hair. She asked me at that time if my hair would be gone when she got home. I told her that I really didn't know how long it would take to fall out. I think she was a bit sad to see my hair gone and just how different I looked. She said she would not have recognized me. In a few minutes, she was OK. We spent the ride home talking about Europe, laughing, and just enjoying being back together! It was wonderful hearing them all laughing and catching up on life.

Just as a woman with breast cancer experiences distress with a cancer recurrence, so too do family members who love and support her. Until this point, Liz's daughter had not seen her mother without her hair. Seeing her mother look so different must have been a shock and a source of sadness; it also likely served as a reality check for Ashley W., who had been away in Europe. Just knowing that the cancer is back is different from seeing visible proof of its recurrence.

No studies exist on how cancer in a parent affects young adults. We know that parenting children younger than 18 years of age when a mother has cancer adds significant stress to the mother (Moore, Rauch, Baer, Pirl, & Muriel, 2015; Park et al., 2015), but there is nothing written about college-aged children and their responses to the diagnosis of cancer in a parent. Although a young adult gains independence when they leave for college, they still are their parents' child and are affected by the cancer, perhaps even more so when they are not there for the daily challenges facing their parent with cancer.

Ashley W. showed us what she brought home from her trip and shared some of her stories. It sounded like her time over there was amazing! She brought me some beautiful scarves that I will be wearing at some point. She brought her stepdad this great chef's hat from Paris. It was exciting.

Time for a nap. Stay tuned.

July 15, 2014
First day of chemotherapy cycle 2

First of all, thank you so much for all of the cards. Keep them coming. The highlight of the day is hearing, "Mail's here!" I love hearing from all of you.

Second, many of you have sent me scarves and other gifts. I'm not at the thank-you stage yet and feel bad not sending cards. I may try to thank you via email instead.

One thing to share now: Shout-out to Lisa for these awesome slippers. They have these removable things that I can heat up in the microwave. They feel amazing on my feet. I'm not sure how she knew my feet are always cold, but these slippers are terrific. Thanks, Lisa. Love you.

Third, Ashley W. and I spent the day at the cancer center. She is so happy to be home and to fuss over me. She was my chauffeur all day. She got a great orientation on maneuvering a wheelchair, especially in some of the tight exam rooms. By the end of the day, she was an expert.

The nurse accessed my port and drew blood for labs. Then I saw Dr. L. He was quite pleased with my progress and felt my liver size had improved by 50%. Amazing! My labs were better, even my liver function tests. Unfortunately, I also have a small tear in the medial meniscus of my right knee. Two days before my discharge, I stretched in bed and felt this burning pain on the left side of my right knee. It has been difficult to walk, so one of the other physicians examined my leg/knee and confirmed the tear. Back to ice, elevation, and being careful not to put too much pressure on it. Ouch, ouch, and still ouch. No more jogging for me for now.

As Dr. L. was going over the details of my progress, Ashley W. started to cry. I told the doctor that she was my youngest child and that I wanted to be here for milestones in her life. He asked Ashley if she was in school, and she explained that she was a senior at Penn State. I also interjected that she was a cheerleader and gushed about her for a few minutes with tears in my eyes, of course. He said that when I am at her graduation, he wants me to take a picture of both of us. I should send it to him, and he will put it on his desk. His assistant, Michele, told me that he really will do that. Wow. Pretty impressive!

We went to the waiting room of the treatment center. They brought a cart around with some soup and a half sandwich. Ashley W. and I both had something, just enough to hold us over. The volunteers managing the cart were so sweet—two older men who had retired a while ago.

We then went into a room in the treatment center for the chemotherapy. The staff, especially the nurses, was terrific. As premedication, I had an IV of two long-acting, antinausea meds. They are supposed to keep the nausea under control for the first 3–5 days. Also, I had dexamethasone. A nurse then gave me doxorubicin and cyclophosphamide as the chemotherapy drugs. Dr. L. decided to switch to this "doublet" after the terrible response I had to the docetaxel and capecitabine. I will use this new regimen for cycle 3 before repeating my scans.

Well, that's it for now. Stay tuned for the side effects. I was very disappointed last time, as I was not properly educated about the side effects. Should the nurse have done that? The physician? The janitor? I know more now from personal experience and am doing my best to prevent the issues I had last time. I am asking more questions specific to the symptoms. Wish me luck.

Educating patients about potential side effects is an important part of nursing care. Patient education allows patients to be an active partner in their care and affords them the opportunity to ask questions and seek clarification about instructions so that potential misunderstandings can be addressed before they become emergencies (Tirodkar et al., 2015). Liz's desire to prevent problems is really good rationale for providing the patient with information/education. For some reason, she did not receive the information that she needed. Her response this time is to ask lots of questions; however, not all patients will ask questions or even know that they need to or can ask questions.

We know that educating patients about what to expect before surgery can improve their knowledge, reduce anxiety, and ultimately, increase their satisfaction with care (Waller et al., 2015). Educating patients about various aspects of pain management can improve what is done about their pain, but this is a complex process that is not solely dependent on the patient (Adam, Bond, & Murchie, 2015). Patient education programs focusing on alleviating fatigue have been shown as beneficial to some (Du et al., 2015). Patient education about symptom clusters may have benefits in improving functional performance (Xiao, Chow, So, Leung, & Chan, 2015). *Symptom clusters* are groups of symptoms that people with cancer experience at the same time that appear to be connected. An example of a symptom cluster is breathlessness, fatigue, and anxiety.

Educating patients about chemotherapy is an important role for nurses. One-on-one sessions with a nurse have been found to be useful, and supplementing these sessions with written material has benefits. Audiovisual materials (e.g., videos, DVDs) and multiple teaching methods can improve retention and may especially be useful for patients with low literacy skills. Outcomes of patient education include better adherence to treatment regimens, improved knowledge about treatment, the need to report side effects in a timely manner instead of waiting for the next appointment, and reduction of patient anxiety (Valenti, 2014). Patient education is not the sole responsibility of the nurse, as pharmacist involvement has been shown to be beneficial (Avery & Williams, 2015).

July 19, 2014

Today is day 4 since cycle 2 started on July 15. So far, the side effects are manageable. I have been trying to eat and drink to keep up my strength. I definitely am tired yet try my best to get up and walk around.

My knee is quite sore, so I have been keeping ice on it intermittently. It has somewhat restricted my movement.

My peeps from work stopped by yesterday afternoon for a while. It was so wonderful to see all of them and just laugh. They certainly brightened my day.

All of the kids are home, including the girls' boyfriends. It is nice to hear all of them in the house, although it certainly is noisier than usual. ☺

I am starting to get nervous about the next week, as that is when I landed in the hospital during cycle 1. I realize that the meds are different this time around, yet that scary feeling still is there. I'm doing my best to stay positive.

Short update this time around. Need a nap. Please continue to send your prayers and positive thoughts. I so appreciate them.

July 21, 2014

Well, I was into week 2 when things crashed and burned during the first cycle. However, I am doing MUCH better this time. My mouth and throat still are sore yet are much more manageable with everything I am doing. I am able to eat and drink to keep up my nutrition. I thank the Lord about 100 times per day for a better outcome this time. The IV meds they gave me before the chemotherapy during cycle 2 also have kept the nausea and vomiting at bay (knock on wood).

The nubs of hair on my head continue to fall out. About one-third of my head is bald so far. It feels really weird, yet I am slowly adjusting to no hair. It certainly is much less prep time after I take a bath. Pat dry and DONE. Many of you have given me scarves and do-rags, which have been greatly appreciated. Shout-out to Rosy today for the new pink (surprise) cap that I am wearing. It is very soft, fits my head well, and fits the back of my head with gentle elastic and two ties hanging down. It also is nice and warm for when I get a bit cold. I plan to get a few more of these for lounging around the house.

I started going through a bunch of journals I had from work. I'm not nearly as anal about saving many of the articles, yet I am at least reviewing them. I am throwing out a lot of the information after I read through it.

Yesterday, we had a really nice family dinner that my husband cooked. I think he has been going through cooking withdrawal, so he made a feast for all of us, including Ashley W.'s boyfriend and some of Patrick's friends. Ashley E.'s boyfriend had to leave early for his five-hour drive back to just outside of Philly. My dad stopped by, and it was nice to spend some time with him and hear about everything he is doing. After a while, he looked a bit tired, so we sent him home with a nice care package of food.

I also did a phone interview for Capella University, where I completed my PhD. They are writing an alumni update article for their magazine. It was exciting to talk about my research and PhD program. I felt my brain kick into gear, which was reassuring. I guess all that daytime TV hasn't completely numbed my brain cells.

Today, I watched a marathon of *Grey's Anatomy*, starting from the very first season on Netflix. It was fun to see the old shows with the original characters. Now, if I could just find *St. Elsewhere*. I was able to purchase the first season on iTunes last year, but I cannot find any other season.

That's all for now. Please continue to send those prayers, as I really think they are helping.

July 26, 2014

I ended up back in the hospital today with a temperature of 102.8°, which meant I was neutropenic again. They started pumping me full of antibiotics. My fever broke, going down to 99.4°.

When they told me they were doing blood cultures, all I could think of was sepsis, which could cause my death. I pictured myself in the intensive care unit (ICU) on a ventilator. Luckily, all was negative. Whew! In my mind, it will be the side effects that will kill me and not the cancer.

July 27, 2014
Still in the hospital

The chills returned and my temperature spiked again after 24 hours in the hospital. This time, they drew more blood cultures and sent my urine for a culture/sensitivity to see if I had an infection.

Everything came back negative after waiting for what seemed like forever. The nurse practitioner was extremely helpful at explaining everything. She told me, "Patients need patience." Good advice!

Today starts day 2 back in the hospital. I was readmitted yesterday for a fever. They checked my counts, and the neutrophils (part of the WBC family) were at 0. So, I again have a neutropenic fever. They are pumping me full of antibiotics and did a second set of blood cultures earlier this morning because I spiked another fever. I'm not sure how long I will be here this time.

This whole situation is so depressing. My birthday is this week, and I was planning to stop by my office on Tuesday to celebrate with the gang. Not sure if that will happen now.

It is disheartening for people to go back and forth from living at home to being admitted to the hospital. For some people, it may get easier because they know what to expect. For others, this is what makes it more difficult. They know what it is like to be in the hospital, and repetition does not make the experience any easier or better! Liz was hoping to celebrate her birthday at home and to see work colleagues; this admission to the hospital put this in jeopardy, making her understandably upset.

Being admitted to the hospital with febrile neutropenia has significant costs to the system; average costs per admission for women with breast cancer range from $11,132 to $37,087 (Dulisse et al., 2013; Pathak et al., 2015). This does not take into account patient costs, including lost income, emotional burden, and intangible costs to their families.

July 28, 2014

I woke up with numbness in my right knee, right fingers, and left fingers. There was no burning or paresthesias. By this point, my hands were peeling, especially between my fingers—side effects of the capecitabine. They sent more blood cultures.

I also had a CT scan of my abdomen and chest with contrast today. I've had so many of these tests because my oncologist wants to keep a close eye on the cancer. I'm nervous about all of the radiation yet realize the cancer will kill me before any radiation side effects.

Dr. L. came to see me and offered to show me the test results. I said "OK," which he was shocked to hear. I think he is learning that I want to see and talk details about everything. He was pleased with the scans.

This evening, my right knee and leg were swollen. The nurse came in and elevated my leg on two pillows. She was concerned about an embolus. (That's a blood clot for those of you not used to this medical jargon.)

July 29, 2014

I had a Doppler appointment first thing in the morning to rule out a deep vein thrombosis. Essentially, they were trying to rule out a blood clot. Thrombus = blood clot. Results were negative, which is good.

A physical therapist came to help me start walking again. I moved from a wheelchair to using a quad cane. We then used a walker to get started and graduated to a regular cane after several trips around the unit. The therapist even had me walking up and down the three steps in the rehab area. I felt so awkward because, again, I had helped people with orthopedic injuries or other needs for rehab in the past. Now, here I was as the patient. The pain in my knees made moving up and down these steps quite a challenge. However, I had to pass this test to get home. It felt strange to walk again, and I was somewhat embarrassed to walk around with these devices. However, I realized that these were tools that would help me get better. It still was amazing how much my legs did not support me walking—all from a week in bed. I cannot imagine how these other patients did it after weeks in the ICU.

It was about this time that I talked to Dr. L. about laser therapy on my mouth, tongue, and cheeks. The mucositis was so painful, and I needed more help to decrease it, which would decrease the pain. He did not approve of this approach. I will try again after I talk with some of my professional contacts.

During the middle of the night, I could not sleep. I turned on the TV, which I thought would make me sleepy. Instead, I somehow landed on the shopping channel and, in my drugged state, started ordering things. Very dangerous! I couldn't even remember what I ordered other than a green lounge chair for me to sit by the pool. It had a canopy, so I would be somewhat protected from the sun. It was my birthday present to myself. Boy, was my husband going to be excited when all this crap started to come to the house. NOT!

July 30, 2014

Dr. L. came into my room a bit angry over this laser therapy thing. He said, "I know you sent out all your spies to talk with me. Just so you know, it doesn't work!"

I kind of chuckled under my breath. I did contact lots of my peeps to work on him, and it seems like they were quite successful. By the end of our visit, he approved the laser treatments and wrote orders for them in my chart. I just wanted him to know that I don't drop the subject that quickly or that easily when I feel strongly about it. Now, that's what I call patient advocacy!

I started the laser treatments later that day. Annette (a certified registered nurse practitioner) came directly to my room several times while I was in the hospital, and I started to feel a little bit better. Annette helped me start methods that would ease the pain and decrease the mucositis. She was incredibly helpful.

Dr. L. and his entourage came back later in the day and said I could go home. Well, I started to cry. Dr. L. asked, "Why are you crying? I just gave you good news!" I told him I was so happy to get home to celebrate my birthday tomorrow. Each time I am admitted to the hospital, I always think of problems in the back of my mind. When I get to go home, I am so grateful.

July 31, 2014
Back home

I was able to celebrate my 58th birthday at home! I've never been so excited about a birthday. It felt wonderful to wake up in my own bed. I got to see my family, and my husband made us all a wonderful dinner. I never take my family and my improvement for granted. I know that I could leave my family any day because of this disease. The whole life and death thing is tough to endure. My next long-term goal is to stay alive to see 59.

This entry perfectly explains the roller coaster nature of cancer. Four days after feeling depressed about being in the hospital, Liz is home and celebrating her birthday. Of course, this is a bittersweet experience for her—the tenuous nature of living with metastatic cancer removes the false certainty that many of us have that there always is another birthday to be celebrated.

August 2, 2014

To recap, I stayed in the hospital until Wednesday, July 30. I suffered with many of the same side effects as the last round of chemotherapy, especially since my neutrophils (type of WBC) dropped to 0 again. I also ended up with serious swelling in my legs from all of the IV fluid. I had to have physical therapy and learn to walk with a cane to get home.

They did repeat CT scans of my chest, abdomen, and pelvis. My oncologist was very pleased with the decrease in cancer in my liver and said we might be able to slightly decrease the dosage of the chemotherapy to help with the side effects. We'll see.

My next treatment was originally scheduled for Tuesday, August 5, but it was rescheduled to Friday, August 8, to give me a few more days to recover from the last treatment. They are going to give me a dose of pegfilgrastim to help my bone marrow produce WBCs. It hopefully will minimize the loss of neutrophils and help prevent some of the side effects. I hope it works.

Pegfilgrastim is a drug that stimulates the production of WBCs to help fight infection. The drug has a number of side effects, including the potential for the spleen to rupture and the development of acute respiratory distress syndrome. Like all medications, there has to be a balance between potential harms and benefits. In this case, Liz is given this medication to prevent infection, as the chemotherapy has destroyed her WBCs.

Today was a continuance of my birthday celebration and my return home. Many of my family and friends stopped by and stayed for dinner. My dad came over and gave me this really pretty scarf with pink hearts on it. He said he went all over to find it. It was so very sweet.

That's all for now. I need to get some sleep. Thanks to all of you for your cards, gifts, and ongoing words of encouragement. I am so very appreciative.

August 11, 2014

I received a dose of pegfilgrastim by subcutaneous injection to help increase my WBCs. I also started on ondansetron, instead of prochlorperazine, for its antinausea effect. The ondansetron is very effective!

August 13, 2014

Today is day 5 of chemotherapy cycle 3. Only two more treatments to go! This time, I received another medication to help my WBCs regenerate after the chemotherapy. The doctor hopes it will keep me out of the hospital. We shall see.

I have been sore and tired from the shot. It feels like the flu with achy bones. I am quite sick of just sitting around all day watching mindless television. However, I realize that rest is the best thing I can do for my body right now, so I am trying to be tolerant.

My Aunt Gail visited for about five days. It was wonderful to have her here to fuss over me and hang out with the family. She went back home yesterday morning.

As many of you may know, we donated Amanda's organs when she died in November 2001. We met the young lady who received Amanda's liver—Dayna Marie—in June 2009. We developed a close relationship with Dayna and her family. She called me "Mommy #2," and I called her "Daughter #3." This past week, she had liver rejection and was put on the transplant list for a second liver. Unfortunately, Dayna died before a second liver was available. We are grateful that Amanda's liver gave Dayna 13 more years of life yet are so sad that she only lived to be 25 years old. Patrick and Ashley W. drove to her home near Detroit, Michigan, for the viewing yesterday and the funeral today. I feel so bad that I could not attend yet am so proud of my kids for representing the Wertz family. Sue, Dayna's mom, allowed us to put a Beanie Babies panda bear in Dayna's casket in memory of Amanda.

Today also is the second anniversary of my mom's death. She sure lived her 80 years to the max, yet I miss her so much every day, especially since I have been sick. I just want to sit beside her with her arm around me while she says everything will be OK. However, I think this chemotherapy and how it has affected me would have been way too much for her. So, I settle for happy memories and her love from heaven.

That's all for now. Keep those prayers coming.

August 16, 2014

I was admitted to the same hospital today for another round of neutropenia. They gave me strong antibiotics and some potassium supplementation for a potassium of 3.0 (that is a low number).

Being an emergency nurse back in the day, I was nervous about having to go to the emergency department, or ED, because of the number of sick patients usually waiting to be seen. My last two admissions were direct to the oncology unit to minimize my exposure to germs. So this time around I wore a mask when we got there and tried not to touch anything. Luckily, it was not very busy that morning, as there were only a few people in the waiting room. We didn't wait very long and were escorted directly to a private room used for isolation. Everyone who came into the room wore a mask, making me feel really safe from any potential germs hanging around. The staff told me that they were used to patients with neutropenia because of the cancer center in this area and the number of people they see going through chemotherapy. Another reason to go directly to this hospital!

The next event was accessing my port. I had been told not to let anyone other than an experienced oncology nurse touch it. So, being the shy person that I am, I asked the nurse in the room about her experience with ports. She said she does them all the time because of the number of patients admitted via the ED from the cancer center. She sounded very positive and like she knew what she was talking about. Therefore, I trusted her and let her access my port. She did a great job, even though she was not the traditional oncology nurse. It goes to show that ICU and ED nurses also see lots of patients with cancer yet do not consider themselves oncology nurses. We need to create more resources for these "nontraditional" cancer nurses.

Earlier tonight, I was starting to get nervous just sitting alone in my bed. I had no idea what they were doing out there. I did not see a nurse from 7:30 pm to 10:45 pm. When a nurse did show up, she told me she was "busy." She did NOT have a very good bedside manner. I was quite disappointed, as I could not trust someone like her. I was getting liquid hydromorphone hydrochloride for my abdominal pain. I diligently checked everything she gave me.

August 18, 2014

My blood work came back today with several items that were not good. My hemoglobin was 7.4 and my hematocrit was 21.6. These numbers are quite low, so I was scheduled to have one unit of blood.

They gave me 25 mg of diphenhydramine before the transfusion and wanted to give me acetaminophen (Tylenol®). I refused it because of the cancer in my liver, even though I had these other drugs in my body being metabolized through my liver. However, this was one drug that I could control.

Me: "Why do you give acetaminophen?"

Nurse: "It's the protocol." (No, I did not choke her! To me, that's like hearing, "It's not my job.")

Me: "What do you want it to do?"

Nurse: "Decrease any fever."

Me: "How about Advil®?"

Nurse: "No, it won't work the same as Tylenol."

Oh boy. I think it would have taken more effort to get the order for Advil, so she blew it off. Pretty sad. I figured it wasn't that big of a deal, so I didn't press the issue. However, I did not take the acetaminophen.

This is a clear example of poor communication between nurse and patient. As a nurse, Liz is aware of the side effects of the drugs she has to take. She does not want to take medication that will put additional strain on her liver, but the nurse is insistent that she take it. A power struggle results that erodes the relationship, which may have consequences in the future for both Liz and the nurse. The nurse may see Liz as a "difficult" patient, labeling her for all future encounters. Liz sees the nurse as uncaring and someone who is not respectful of her as a person with knowledge of her body and agency over her care. The nurse discounted Liz's concerns, and as a result, Liz did not take the medication. The medication was not a life-saving one, but what if it was essential and Liz did not take it?

Communication is a central aspect of the nurse–patient relationship. Patients are highly sensitive to various aspects of the communication process and often are dissatisfied with this process. Good communication comforts, supports, and guides the patient toward the best outcome possible. Poor communication makes the patient feel demeaned and distressed (Thorne, Oliffe, Oglov, & Gelmon, 2013). Nurses often are rushed to do the work they need to do. Patients are aware of this and will make excuses for lack of attention or presence (McCabe, 2004). While the patient may find communication problematic, nurses also are frustrated by their inability to make time to talk to patients—problems exacerbated by understaffing and workload pressures (Watts, Botti, & Hunter, 2010).

Some healthcare providers listen more effectively to their patients and are perceived as more empathetic; nurses tend to do better in this aspect of care than oncologists (Finset, Heyn, & Ruland, 2013). However, oncology care providers often act in isolation with little team cohesion. This influences patient care when a lack of confidence exists in what the patient has been told and by whom. Nurses may be reluctant to seek clarification, and the end result is that the patient suffers (Chen & Raingruber, 2014; Wittenberg-Lyles, Goldsmith, & Ferrell, 2013).

Sometimes I feel like a "secret shopper," yet instead of being in a department store, I am in the hospital. And the merchandise is ME! I have seen some great nurses and physicians yet also have seen what is wrong with our healthcare system.

Around 1:15 pm, the blood for the transfusion arrived at the unit. The nurse was running around trying to find a second RN to sign off before the transfusion. She came into my room and hung the bag on an IV pole while she was getting everything ready. I looked up to make sure she would be running it through saline. She was.

I was quite nervous, as I had never had a blood transfusion. I had administered blood to many patients during my active nursing days and had seen major reactions. Yes, another case of "I knew too much." I asked if I could see the bag. The nurse was quite confused and said, "The bag is hanging right here."

I asked to see the label and told her it was nothing personal against her. I checked my name, blood type, expiration date, etc. I told her the same thing—that I had done all this research on patient safety and quality and just wanted to be sure I was getting the right unit. She said, "Oh, I understand. We make mistakes all the time."

Uggggghhhhhh!!!

Just what I wanted to hear. Such a common, accepting attitude instead of Dr. Peter Pronovost's goal to get to ZERO errors. I sat there and waited for some type of reaction but nothing happened. Good news. Between the diphenhydramine and the hydromorphone I had for pain, I slept through most of the transfusion.

Patients have every right to check medications and IV infusions; potentially dangerous substances are going into their body, and they have a right to ask about these and to participate in ensuring accuracy. Patients can act as a check on the safety of administration. They should look at the label on the IV bag and ensure that it is their name and date of birth. Merely asking the patient's name to ensure that it is the right patient is not necessarily accurate; patients may not hear correctly, may be drowsy, and may answer "yes," even if they did not hear correctly. Many procedures require the nurse to check the patient information on the medication or infusion against the patient's identification bracelet or bar code.

As a nurse and a patient, it is very frustrating to not have control of your own care. I am such a perfectionist. After five years of research on quality of care, medical errors, and electronic health records, I want to contribute to my care and not just be a room number, such as "Room 608 wants something for pain." That type of communication is so degrading. I know I did that as a clinical nurse. I got to see for myself how it feels to just be a number.

To cap off the day, I requested something for pain at 10 pm. I heard nothing until 10:45 pm, when she brought in the liquid pain reliever. She kept apologizing for being so late.

Liz clearly feels frustrated. She wants to be treated as a person, not a disease or room number. As a nurse, she wants recognition that she has nursing knowledge as well as knowledge of herself as an individual. *Person-centered care* refers to an approach taken to patient care that is respectful of the individual as a unique person, offers choices to the patient based on his or her wishes, and allows for negotiation of care (Morgan & Yoder, 2012).

Another way of looking at person-centered care is offered by Richardson (2004), who describes it as the following:

· Responding to the individual needs of the person with cancer

· Recognizing the central role of the family and their support needs

· Caring that extends over the course of the illness, meeting a broad range of needs

· Valuing the knowledge, skills, and resources that the patient and family possess

· Involving the patient in the planning process

· Caring that is culturally sensitive

August 19, 2014

The same thing happened this morning. I was supposed to get my pain meds at 6:30 am. I was told that my nurse was not available. I understood that this was possibly change of shift, yet SOMEONE should have told me SOMETHING. I ended up getting the drug at 8:10 am. Not acceptable! I started to get nervous around medication time. We were trying to get into a rhythm where we stayed ahead of the pain. That clearly was not working. I was incredibly frustrated.

Pain control is extremely important, as delaying a dose of medication can lead to the pain getting out of control. It is a basic tenet of pain control that medication be given at regular intervals (Swarm et al., 2013), with additional medication if the patient is experiencing breakthrough pain (pain that occurs despite regular medication) (Caraceni et al., 2013). Breakthrough pain is common in patients with advanced cancer and causes significant distress to patients and their family.

I was discharged this afternoon and left the hospital around 3:30 pm. Good thing, because I was getting ready to really cause a fuss. Maybe it was the psychological boost of getting to go home or perhaps the blood transfusion, but I felt like I had more energy today. I actually felt good! Ashley W. and Ashley E. came to pick me up. It was so great to get outside, feel the sun on my face (yes, it stopped raining for me), smell the fresh air, and ride in the car. Woo-hoo. What a good day!

Liz had anemia, a common occurrence after chemotherapy. This lack of red blood cells affects energy level and general well-being, as these cells carry oxygen to all parts of the body. Low red cells means less oxygen, so replacing those cells with a blood transfusion means that the patient's blood will have more oxygen. The boost of energy that results makes people feel much better.

August 20, 2014

Today was my husband's birthday. I felt energetic, so we all went to the Pittsburgh Pirates baseball game to celebrate. We borrowed a wheelchair from a good friend of ours because my legs were still very weak. They pushed me all around, even though I felt very embarrassed being in a chair. My husband had contacted the Pirates' offices to make sure we were all set. The disability office was terrific in helping us. Even the staff around our seats was so helpful. I was a very satisfied customer.

It was a good game! The Pirates actually won, which broke a six-game losing streak. It was wonderful to be out at the park and to spend quality time with my family. Patrick met us at the game before going back to school.

That's all for now. Keep those prayers coming. They are definitely helping. God is good!

August 21, 2014

I've stopped going to get my laser treatments for the mucositis. My mouth is healing nicely, and I am tired of making that trip three days per week. Now that I'm discharged, I would have to drive to the hospital for every treatment. That comes to three times per week for a 10-minute treatment each day. The hospital is approximately 45 minutes from my home. It's a major trip considering I have to find someone to take me, as I am not back to driving. My husband already has missed a lot of work, so I've been leaning on friends to take turns being my chauffeur. Annette, the nurse giving me the treatments, did everything she could to support me and made the appointments whenever I could get there. That time frame doesn't include a doctor's visit once per week.

Whew! I was a busy gal. But I was just getting the help I needed for that nasty mucositis. Dr. L. told me that what I had was a level 4 mucositis, which I was told was the most serious.

Attending multiple appointments every week for extended periods of time is not unusual for people with cancer. As with Liz, the distances can be long and the time away from home, friends, and family significant. This adds to the burden of disease, especially the expense and inconvenience to both the patients and the people who drive them to and from appointments. Some institutions offer navigation services (lay or nurse navigators) to help patients with transportation needs.

August 25, 2014

Today, all of the kids went back to school. We have one at Duquesne University, one at Indiana University of Pennsylvania, and one at Penn State University. They are all seniors!

The house is so quiet with all of them gone. I miss them terribly when they are at school. I'm also very proud of all of them for graduating this year. Those tuition expenses are brutal! On top of three college tuition payments, we have all the expenses related to my medical needs.

August 28, 2014

Today, I went to my office for a visit. A colleague at ONS picked me up at 9:30 am and drove me to the office. One of the girls pushed me around in a wheelchair. It was VERY hard to give in and let someone push me around. However, I could not walk that far in the office. That continues to be an issue for me—to let people help me. I always have been an independent person and have always helped SOMEONE ELSE!

I stayed in the office from 10 am to 1 pm. It was fabulous to see everyone. My peeps at the office laid down the rules for everyone. They reserved one of our training rooms for people to come visit me and decorated it in pink. It really worked out well. So many staff members stopped in to see me, bringing all kinds of pink goodies. Our current CEO gave me a hug and wished me good luck. She is retiring from her role soon. Our new CEO is starting in September. She was in town to get the transition started. I already knew her from other projects. When she saw me, she gave me a genuine hug that I could tell came from her heart. It really felt great. I will be reporting to her when I go back to work.

One of the biggest challenges for some people when they are ill is to let go of control and let others help them. Liz is no exception! Her colleagues, many of them with experience in oncology nursing, created a plan to maximize her ability to see her workplace friends by providing her with a space (decorated in pink for breast cancer support) where she could meet and greet them. This was a thoughtful and caring gesture.

August 30, 2014

Ashley W. is in her senior year at Penn State. Today, she is in Ireland, cheering in a different time zone. We had a bunch of adults and kids here to enjoy swimming. We had the radio on listening to the football game; Penn State won in the last minute. I sat outside most of the afternoon. Because I am supposed to stay out of the sun, I was in a shaded area.

I also had some time to talk with Marvin, my brother-in-law, who happens to be a pastor. We talked a lot about my cancer and my reaction to it. I really am afraid to die. We also discussed some positive things I can do to get through this feeling.

Most of the attention of research on the causes of distress for women with breast cancer focuses on early breast cancer and the experiences of women in the first two years after diagnosis. Little attention is paid to women living with metastatic cancer (Butler et al., 2003). Fear of dying is a known source of distress for these women. This fear can take many forms: the process of dying itself and not knowing if there will be pain, loss of control, being a burden to others, and suffering at the end of life. There also is the fear associated with not being a part of the family anymore and leaving behind loved ones (Kenne Sarenmalm, Thorén-Jönsson, Gaston-Johansson, & Öhlén, 2009). Women often are not able to be open with others about these fears (Vilhauer, 2008), partially because they want to protect family and friends from their suffering. Fear of dying has been shown to occur in 69% of women with metastatic breast cancer (Mayer, 2010).

Factors contributing to distress for these women include the uncertainty of living with noncurable cancer, lack of control of the situation, and poor emotional functioning (depression and anxiety) (Warren, 2010). Not being able to continue with normal daily activities and dealing with physical symptoms of the disease and side effects of treatment are also contributors to poor emotional quality of life (Mosher et al., 2013).

How women prepare for their own death is deeply personal, but some commonalities exist, as identified in a 2008 study of women with metastatic breast cancer (Chunlestskul, Carlson, Koopmans, & Angen, 2008). Women reported that their preparations for death were related to the experiences they had of others in their family dying. These women worried that their deaths would be devastating for those they would leave behind. This was a source of guilt for some. The women recognized that they needed to prepare for their eventual deaths, that this would take time, and that they could not do it alone. Women said that talking about their death was uncomfortable for others and they felt silenced because of this. When they did bring death up, family members sometimes acted in ways that were hurtful or as if talking about death would make it happen, which would end any attempts to discuss it.

Liz reached out to her brother-in-law, a pastor, for help with this existential crisis. Being a woman of faith, she seeks comfort within her religion.

August 31, 2014

Today, we had people here to swim and barbeque and really had a nice day. I did not swim, but it was nice to be outside with everyone. My dad came over today, and we all had a great conversation. My son Patrick said that was the first time he heard his PapPap talk so much. They talked about religion, wars, and fighter planes over the last two weekends he has been over! See, the old guy still has it! He is 84 years old now and was 82 when my mom died in August 2012. We pay for a lot of his expenses, yet he STILL has a part-time job delivering auto parts because he wants to be independent and contribute something to cover some of his expenses.

We used to invite him over for dinner on Sundays all the time. Most of the time, he wouldn't come over. He builds and flies radio-controlled airplanes and spent most of his time then flying them at the local airplane club. Now, he comes over every Sunday. Since I have been sick, he tries to come over to see me or lets me know if he can't.

My dad just wants to check on me to make sure I am OK. He usually doesn't talk too much. This relapse has told me that he is worried about me, so he makes these visits. He also says that he loves me and lets me kiss him on the lips.

I think he changed when my mom died.

He does not want to be left out of the information loop. He stops by whenever he can, and it does make me feel better. I would love for him to hold me. He didn't do that much when I was a kid. He worked three jobs when I was young to keep our family on track.

No matter how old a parent's child is, the parent will be concerned about the child's health and well-being. Liz's father exemplifies this in his actions. He visits more frequently and obviously worries about her health. Beach and White (2013) address this in their book about parents helping their seriously ill adult child. They talk about the need for boundaries, the ability of people to change past behaviors and overcome decades of poor communication, and how parents can help their ill adult child instrumentally, emotionally, and financially (if possible).

In just a few sentences, Liz describes how her father is giving her the love and attention that she craved when she was younger—things that he couldn't provide because he was so busy. It is a poignant description of love and healing and our ability to change, even when we are older.

September 3, 2014

I had yet another PET/CT to check on everything inside of me. It is such a process! You have to drink this disgusting drink—two of them! Then, you have to wait an hour in a dark room (on purpose) to slow your metabolism. You are not permitted to text (my children could NEVER stop texting!), read, etc. They want you to be completely rested for this test. In fact, one time I was so relaxed that I fell asleep! The technician told me that many patients have fallen asleep in the past. After, you have to wait another 50 minutes for the radioactive material to get through your body.

September 6, 2014

We drove up to Penn State to watch Ashley W. cheer at a home football game. It was wonderful to go. I slept off and on during the three-hour drive. We got a hotel room, which was not too far from the stadium.

I was so nervous traveling because I had not been this far from home since the recurrence. I took my meds with me. My husband goes through them each morning and evening so that I take the right meds at the right time. (Hmm, that sounds like a nursing thing.)

What I was most worried about was the pain. I was taking hydrocodone hydrochloride liquid by mouth to address the pain while I was at home. It makes me very tired. After what we went through with my first hospitalization, I did not want to go into panic mode. This issue probably is my biggest concern.

I also was wondering about regular food. There weren't many healthy foods at the concession stands. I was having nausea and vomiting, making me afraid that I would throw up at my seat. I did have my antinausea drugs, ondansetron and prochlorperazine, with me and took them every six to eight hours, as directed. The prochlorperazine made me sleepy. I did not want to sleep during the game!

I needed to take in some of my meds, a drink, and high-energy protein bars into the stadium. I wasn't so sure what was permitted.

They were selling plastic Penn State clear bags, which were used to bring anything into the stadium. They started to sell these last year as a security measure. So, I shoved everything I had into that clear bag and covered up some of the meds with a big sports drink bottle. I put the bag on my lap and we went through the entrance gate (in a separate line). No one even looked at the bag. We were escorted to the elevator. Everyone was so unbelievable!

The staff at Penn State was amazing! My husband got in touch with people in their separate Office for Disability Services by browsing the university's website. They are very, very accommodating to anyone with a disability. They had a large, separate parking area with buses going back and forth to the stadium. I would never have been able to walk all that way, especially on those cold, windy days. We had our game tickets and our disability tag, so we were set to go. I was surprised and impressed that there were so many people who had special needs. In fact, I wanted to help some other older people who looked sicker—typical nurse!

There was an elevator with two police officers and a separate entrance. We used it for several games. Even though I hated being in that wheelchair, I felt like a princess for getting all of this attention. We got to our seats, and the usher talked with my husband and stored the wheelchair for us. At the end of the game, she got out the wheelchair and had it ready for us. I was so impressed with their customer service.

Later in the evening was the Parents and Family Weekend Banquet at Nittany Lion Inn in the Mount Nittany Room. Ashley W. sat with us, and we got to meet some of the other cheerleaders and their families.

September 8, 2014

Today is my seventh wedding anniversary. My husband has been so terrific taking care of me without any reward for his actions. I'm sure he thinks that he did not sign up for this mess, and I feel terrible for what HE is going through. His first wife had several medical issues and died at the young age of 42. My second husband was killed in a car crash and also died at 42.

I think Hipp and I thought we were heading into a stable relationship without any medical trauma. I keep apologizing for not being there for him. He pushes off the bad news and focuses on the positive news. He has been my "Rock of Gibraltar."

Cancer is regarded as a couple's disease. Couples tend to cope with and react to the disease both as individuals and as a couple; this is called *dyadic coping*. Very few studies exist on couples where the woman has metastatic cancer. Like many other studies on women with breast cancer, the focus is on women with early-stage disease. It has been shown that couples coping with metastatic breast cancer continue to act as primary supports for each other. This is seen as a good thing, as it is similar to the way many couples deal with everyday normal challenges—by being mutually supportive. When the woman with breast cancer and her partner/spouse cope well with the challenges of living with cancer, their mutual adjustment is better. However, if they cope negatively, it affects both of them negatively, too (Badr, Carmack, Kashy, Cristofanilli, & Revenson, 2010).

How the partner/spouse copes also is partially dependent on his or her past experiences with loss. Living with metastatic cancer is an ongoing threat. How the partner deals with protracted stress is an important factor in the amount of stress/distress experienced (Butler et al., 2005). Liz and her husband both have experienced the loss of a spouse in the past. This undoubtedly influences their experience of Liz's illness.

September 10, 2014

I apologize for the delay in getting a new update to you. Fortunately, the news has been mostly good. I had a PET scan done on September 3 and saw my oncologist on September 9. He was quite pleased with the results and said the cancer was decreasing as a result of the chemotherapy drugs. GREAT NEWS! Starting on September 3, I was able to walk into the cancer center instead of using a wheelchair. Very invigorating for me!

He also changed my treatment regimen from "high and hard" to "low and long." As you know, I ended up in the hospital after each of the three chemotherapy treatments. He was giving me high doses of the drugs, which caused lots of side effects, including the neutropenia that caused my hospital admissions. So, now he is giving me small amounts of doxorubicin over a longer period of time to decrease the side effects and give my body a bit of a rest. My quality of life also is supposed to improve because of the decreased side effects.

Maintaining a balance between the effectiveness of treatment and the patient's quality of life is more art than science. Intense chemotherapy leads to side effects that not only affect quality of life but pose a threat to life itself. Every time Liz's WBCs fell to low levels, it put her at risk for infection. Her mouth ulcers also were a result of intense chemotherapy. Switching to another approach—low and long—is an effort to control the cancer while allowing her body to recover. She also will feel better at home. With less side effects, she may be able to do more.

As of September 9, I now get the doxorubicin once every week for three weeks and then get one week off. This schedule will continue for three months, leading to another PET scan around the beginning of December. At first, I was quite upset about the thought of getting this poison every week. Once I had time to think about it and review details with my life coach (you know who you are!), I am feeling better about the new regimen.

Patients don't always respond well to a change of medication. Some people may think that with the reduced intensity of chemotherapy, the cancer will not be under control. Liz has an opinion about the medication she is getting and sees it as a "poison." It is challenging to allow a "poison" into your body every week. However, Liz thought about it, talked to a trusted confidant, and changed her way of thinking.

The doc and the nurse told me that there would be less side effects. However, this week I had a brutal day on Wednesday, throwing up all day and experiencing piercing pain in my epigastric area (stomach). It was horrendous, and I was SO pissed because I haven't had nausea and vomiting since my first round of chemotherapy. They did not give me the same antinausea medicine as part of the treatment. Well, for my next treatment on Tuesday, September 16, you can bet I will be demanding—yes, demanding—that I get the long-acting antinausea drug before the treatment. I can be a real pain in the ass when I feel strongly about something. Oh, wait, many of you already knew that!

I started taking ondansetron as soon as I could keep anything down. It is an antinausea drug that I can take every eight hours. I am not taking any more chances. I feel a lot better today and can actually eat/drink. In fact, we are going to the Pirates game tonight if I feel up to it. They are playing the Cubs. After the game, there is a Lynyrd Skynyrd concert on the field. Oh boy.

A medication change resulted in renewed side effects because the same supportive medications were not given with the chemotherapy. *Supportive medications* are those that prevent or treat side effects associated with treatment. These include antinausea medications and drugs to promote the production of both white and red blood cells; Liz has received all of these as part of her treatment regimen.

Healthcare providers and patients don't always assess symptoms the same way. In one study, nurses and oncologists overestimated how many of their patients experienced nausea and vomiting as a side effect of chemotherapy. On the contrary, they underestimated the effects of these symptoms on the daily lives of their patients (Vidall et al., 2015).

If I can get adjusted to this new schedule, I hope to go back to work on perhaps a part-time basis. I still am quite tired, so I will have to gradually increase my workload instead of jumping in full speed—difficult for me to do. I plan to meet with our new CEO and discuss some options. I need to understand her expectations.

Work is an important part of "ordinary" life. Liz is starting to think about this, an indication that she is beginning to think about life beyond cancer. There are many different factors that influence whether survivors can go back to work and effectively contribute, including the type of treatment they have received, daily job duties, their mental health, their insurance coverage, their quality of life, and the attitude of their employer. Survivors of breast cancer have the highest return-to-work rate of any of the cancers (93%), but this is for women who have early breast cancer (Islam et al., 2014).

That's all for now. Again, thanks so much for the cards and the goodies that show up in my mailbox. I love hearing from everyone. Oh, and keep those prayers coming. I keep telling God that I'm not done yet with this life! So far, He is listening.

October 10, 2014

For those of you on the East Coast, I hope you are keeping warm with the change in temperature. Fall is officially here. In fact, the end of summer was bittersweet for me. This nightmare started in May, right as summer was beginning. Some of the worst times were over the summer. I'm glad those days are over, yet I already miss the warm weather and sunshine. I need some beach time!

My new chemotherapy regimen is working well. The weekly treatments are less toxic to my body because it is one drug and a lower dose. I'm still tired but not as washed out as those first treatments made me feel. However, I did develop those frickin' mouth ulcers, which made it almost impossible for me to swallow. YUCK! They are starting to go away (finally).

I went to the cancer center this past Tuesday for my weekly treatment. The doctor was very positive about my progress. His words were quite reassuring for me. However, my WBC count was too low, so I did not get chemotherapy this week. I have noticed that my eyelashes and eyebrows are starting to grow back without any chemotherapy for two weeks. That's a good sign.

Keep your prayers coming. I believe they are working!

October 14, 2014

I had a lower dose of chemotherapy today (75% of the previous dose), even though my platelets still were low. I just have to be careful with bumps, bruises, or cuts, as I may bleed longer.

I was so nervous today because it has been two weeks without any chemotherapy. I want it to all be over (just the chemotherapy) yet am still afraid of the side effects. I received palonosetron and dexamethasone intravenously before the chemotherapy to minimize nausea and vomiting. This combination has worked well previously. My husband and sister were there with me, which really helped.

So far, so good. I took a nap. Now, I'm relaxing and watching TV.

Thanks to everyone for your cards, love, prayers, and support—especially now that so much time has gone by. It has been five months already, which is so hard to believe. I still have at least six treatments to go, which will be spread over the next two months.

I am so grateful to my family and all of my friends. Your caring words and love have been such tremendous support and have really helped me get back on my feet when I am feeling sad.

October 22, 2014

Well, another week is going by. I went to the cancer center on Tuesday for my chemotherapy, but my platelets were too low. They were low last week and dropped again. So, there will be no chemotherapy for this warrior princess this week. I'm off until next Tuesday. I'm disappointed, yet I understand the reason for holding it. I'm just anxious to get the chemotherapy treatments behind me.

Because chemotherapy affects many different components of the blood, care is taken to ensure that the levels of these components are safe for additional chemotherapy. This time, Liz's platelets were low. Platelets are involved in clotting. If her blood can't clot, Liz is at risk of bleeding, which can cause further complications.

It is disappointing for patients to have treatment withheld. On one hand, they want their chemotherapy treatment to be over so that they can start to recover and get back to their life. On the other, not having a scheduled chemotherapy treatment can raise fears that the cancer is not being controlled.

October 23, 2014

Today, I went back to work! I am planning on doing one day in the office and one day at home. I didn't get there until 11:30 am, although

I planned on getting there at 10. I had so much trouble doing my hair! Ha ha! No hair certainly decreases the prep time. I actually was trying on clothes and trying to figure out what to wear. All of my pants are so baggy because I have lost almost 25 pounds. I wanted to lose a few pounds but NOT THIS WAY! I don't want to buy new clothes just yet, as I'm not too sure where my weight will end up.

Involuntary weight loss is a significant problem in individuals with cancer. Some people may joke about the "cancer diet." In particular, women may "enjoy" the weight loss, especially if they have struggled with being overweight before cancer. However, weight loss associated with cancer is not a good thing for most survivors, as it may lead to worse outcomes (Mariani, Lo Vullo, & Bozzetti, 2012). In one study of 1,556 survivors, weight loss was 7.1% on average, with 38% having lost more than 10% of their baseline weight (Mariani et al., 2012). In another study, 59% of survivors of cancer had lost at least 10% of their precancer weight and were noted to have poor body image, depression, and decreased sexual interest and satisfaction (Rhondali et al., 2013).

It was so wonderful to see everyone! Today was our "trick-or-treat" day, when staff bring in their kids dressed in Halloween costumes. Most departments have a table with goodies, and the kids go around and stock up on candy. It's kind of a dry run for the real Halloween. The kids were so darned cute!

I was nervous about going back—not sure why. Once I got there and had such a terrific reception from the staff, I felt better. Everyone was so kind and told me how much they missed me. It felt fabulous just sitting in my office and doing something "ordinary," which I had not done since May. I changed the calendars in my office, as they were still all on May. I will be going back in on Friday, as our board will be in town for a meeting.

Returning to work for survivors of cancer often is emotional. They may not be sure of the reception they will receive or how they will be treated moving forward. They may be concerned about their ability to function in the work setting and whether physical or cognitive limitations will affect their ability to work as they did before (Nilsson, Olsson, Wennman-Larsen, Petersson, & Alexanderson, 2011). Women feel vulnerable and insecure about their ability to function in the workplace after cancer. It takes mental preparation to go back to work (Tiedtke, de Rijk, Donceel, Christiaens, & de Casterlé, 2012).

I definitely stayed too long, as I was whipped by 4 pm. Everyone kept telling me to go home. Of course, I didn't listen. ☺ I finally left around 4:30 pm. I fell asleep on the way home and drifted into another lane. My side view mirror scraped another car's side view mirror. It woke me up right away! We each pulled over to the side of the highway and talked. The driver was a nice guy. He had two very small scrapes on his mirror and told me not to worry about it. I didn't even have to use the "C" card. Oh, wait, perhaps the scarf on my head gave away my medical condition!

I was good driving to work but just so tired driving home. On Friday, I am going back to the office with a colleague who lives near me. She will be my chauffeur for the day. Thank you!

This is a good example of Liz overdoing things and not being aware of how tiring this first day back at work would be. Fatigue is a major factor in a successful back-to-work transition. Despite her earlier statement about a graduated process, Liz stayed the whole day! Women who have chemotherapy as part of their treatment report lower vitality and poorer physical health than those who do not (Barnes, Robert, & Bradley, 2014). Liz still is in active treatment. No wonder she's exhausted!

Well, that's enough for now. I'm currently watching our Pittsburgh Penguins play against those pesky Philadelphia Flyers. (That's hockey for those of you who are not sports fans.) The score is tied at 2 with about three minutes left in the second period.

Keep the prayers coming!

October 31, 2014

Happy Halloween to all!

For those of you in the east, dress warm for trick-or-treating tonight and take an umbrella.

I had my chemotherapy treatment this past Tuesday. Again, my platelets were low—even lower than last time. So, the doctor reduced the chemotherapy dose to 10 mg. I questioned the dosage—is it even worth it for just 10 mg? I was told that some chemotherapy is better than no chemotherapy. I will be off next week (no chemotherapy) and then get back onto the three-week regimen. Good thing I can handle last-minute changes. I just want to be done with the chemotherapy and have my body back.

My eyebrows and eyelashes have grown back already. Very exciting! I also have some hair poking through on my head. Woo-hoo! I wore mascara this week for the first time in five months. See, it's the little things that I can celebrate. I guess with some weeks off of the chemotherapy, my body is trying to come back.

I went to work on Wednesday this week; it felt great to be back in the office. I even had one meeting! However, I was quite nauseous and threw up twice. How attractive is that? My colleague was so understanding when I politely excused myself from our meeting, which I greatly appreciated. Whew. I made it through the day. Another colleague who lives nearby was my driver. Thanks to her!

Liz is working while dealing with the side effects of chemotherapy treatment. She is fortunate that she works in a supportive environment with nurses and others who are aware of the issues related to having cancer. Employer attitude plays an important role in successful return-to-work efforts; supportive work environments facilitate return to work. However, some workplaces are hostile, with both employers and coworkers treating the survivor with disrespect. These workplaces deny survivors the work adjustments required to fulfill their job responsibilities (Banning, 2011). Employers may see more barriers to the survivor returning to work than the survivor does, leading to problems during return-to-work planning, as the discrepancy between employer and employee may lead to conflict (Grunfeld, Low, & Cooper, 2010).

Adjustments can be made to the workplace environment and to the way that work is done. These include adjusting the survivor's work schedule so that they work during the hours that they have the most energy, asking the survivor to perform fewer tasks or changing the kind of work that is done, using cognitive prompts for tasks that previously were done using memory, and reducing nonwork activities while at work, such as not using energy to go out for lunch (Sandberg, Strom, & Arcury, 2014).

I rested yesterday and today to get some energy back. We are driving to State College tomorrow to see Ashley W. cheer at the Penn State vs. Maryland football game. I can't wait to see her. The game starts at noon. It is supposed to rain or maybe snow, so I'm not sure how long I will last. We will see Ashley after the game and get something to eat before we go back home.

November 17, 2014

I have been delinquent in posting my updates, so here ya go!

I had a treatment last Tuesday and have another one scheduled for tomorrow. My oncologist was very happy with the physical examination because some of the swelling in my abdomen has gone down. He asked me if I would like "no more chemotherapy" as a Christmas present. I said, "OF COURSE!" Tuesday, November 25, may be my last chemotherapy treatment. Woo-hoo!

I will have another PET scan early in the morning on December 9. At least it is not the 10th, which is the anniversary of my previous husband's death. The doctor will look at the scan on the same day and review the details with me at an appointment later that day. It will be awesome not to have to wait a week to find out. Keep praying!

I have been feeling better since the chemotherapy doses have been lowered. In fact, my hair, eyelashes, and eyebrows are growing back already. It feels so good to see my hair coming in. My scalp is very itchy, as those little pieces of hair keep popping up.

I have been back to work for a few days here and there. I am starting with one day per week. My colleague still is my carpool buddy. I'll be back in the office this Wednesday. I also do some work from home.

My only major side effect is exhaustion. I am so very tired and know that the evidence says to exercise. However, I am too tired to exercise (for you oncology nurses—sound familiar?). I do get exercise on the days we are at the football games and then take a nap on the ride home.

OK, I gotta run. I'll try to post something earlier than a week after my treatment. Until then, keep the prayers coming!

As Liz notes, exercise is an important intervention for reducing treatment-related fatigue (or exhaustion). However, it often feels counterintuitive to exercise when you are tired! Women with breast cancer know that exercise has physical and psychosocial benefits, but there are many barriers to getting the recommended amount of physical activity. These include physical factors (generally related to treatment side effects), environmental factors (e.g., bad weather, lack of time), and psychosocial factors (e.g., lack of social support, lack of motivation) (Brunet, Sabiston, & Burke, 2013). Physical activity during treatment has benefits, including functional improvements such as less fatigue and a feeling of physical empowerment (Backman, Browall, Sundberg, & Wengström, 2016). Exercising also may move the focus from being ill to being healthy and being seen by others as "ordinary" and not "the patient with cancer."

November 20, 2014

Well, I am having a good week. I had my chemotherapy on Tuesday. Thank you, Felicia, for coming with me and my sister Patty for being there, too! So far, so good. I went to work on Wednesday and was there for a full eight hours. Thank you to my colleague for being my carpool partner. It felt wonderful! It is really invigorating being back at work and having to really think again. My brain still works! It is just a bit slow for now.

Cognitive changes often are reported by survivors of breast cancer—described as "brain fog" or "chemo brain." It often is associated with chemotherapy and initially was thought to occur for about six months after treatment and then resolve. However, some women experience these changes for a year following the end of chemotherapy (Collins, 2013). MRI studies have shown a reduction in gray matter in the brain, most often in the frontal and temporal lobes (Lepage et al., 2014).

Women report a variety of changes, including short- and long-term memory loss, problems with attention and concentration, slower processing of information, language difficulties, and problems with executive functioning, such as decision making (Von Ah, Habermann, Carpenter, & Schneider, 2013). These are frustrating and embarrassing and contribute to problems when returning to work.

My eyebrows and eyelashes have grown back in AND my dark hair is growing in. It looks so crazy yet is such a great thing for me to see. It signals that this treatment (and all those yucky side effects) is coming to an end. It feels great!

I am going to Harrisburg this Saturday to present the annual Amanda E. Wertz Memorial EMS for Children Award. I give it every year. This year will be even more special after all I have gone through in 2014. I feel very blessed to be well enough to give the award in person. Patrick and Ashley W. are going with me.

That's all for now. Keep those prayers coming.

November 27, 2014
Thanksgiving

Well, I had my last chemotherapy treatment (I think) on Tuesday of this week. It seemed kind of anticlimactic. In fact, I was done early; we left around 2:30 pm. Now, I have two weeks off and then a PET scan on December 9 at 7:45 am. The doctor will review the results with us later that day.

I am so thankful for all of you who have helped me through this nightmare. I appreciate your cards, gifts, and prayers as I make this journey. Thank you so much.

Happy Thanksgiving to you and your families.

December 12, 2014

I had an appointment with my oncologist on Tuesday of this week. Before the appointment, I had a CT scan and blood work, which he reviewed with me. I'm still neutropenic and anemic. Can you say, "I am frickin' tired all of the time!"

My doctor also wants me to have four more chemotherapy treatments and then see him on January 27 (my brother's birthday). I have one treatment two days before Christmas. That SUCKS! I was so discouraged when he said I would need a few more chemotherapy treatments. I am waiting for a copy of the CT results to try to understand why I have to have more chemotherapy.

On December 9, I left the cancer center and met people from our executive team at work for a holiday luncheon at a restaurant near my office. My husband dropped me off and one of the girls took me home. It was nice.

This week, I was in the office Monday and Thursday. I stayed home on Wednesday, December 10, to feel sorry for myself. I lay in bed until 2 pm. The anniversary of Pat's death and the need for more chemotherapy just got to me. I feel better after my pity party.

There is an overwhelming focus on being positive in cancer survivorship messaging. Women often feel that they have to "think positive" to achieve a good outcome (Wilkinson & Kitzinger, 2000). However, this denies the reality of the many women with metastatic cancer who face a far more uncertain future. Women living with metastatic cancer experience anxiety and depression, sadness, hopelessness, and a fear of the future (Meisel et al., 2012). This is not a sign of weakness but a reality given the nature of the disease. Recognizing feelings and dealing with them is a better strategy than denying them and not dealing with them; Liz had her "pity party" and then felt better.

Depression and anxiety have been shown to persist long after the diagnosis of breast cancer (Mehnert & Koch, 2008). At four years after diagnosis, 38% of women reported moderate to high levels of anxiety and 22% had moderate to high levels of depression.

On Thursday, I was in the office for a few hours in the morning. Later in the day, we went to a hotel for a holiday luncheon for all staff. It was very nice. I was very tired when I got home and took a short nap while watching TV.

I have an echocardiogram on Monday and start chemotherapy on Tuesday. I guess I also should make some time to do some Christmas shopping.

Merry Christmas and happy holidays to all of you. I hope you enjoy the time with your friends and family.

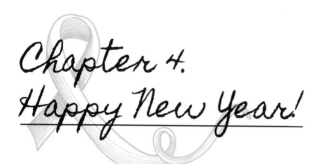

Chapter 4.
Happy New Year!

February 7, 2015

Happy New Year to you and yours!

I apologize for not writing sooner. I have lots to share with you.

Christmas was very nice. All of the kids were home, and we exchanged gifts. We then went to my sister's house for dinner and to exchange more gifts with my family. I rescheduled my chemotherapy for this week so I wouldn't have a ton of side effects on Christmas. I certainly was quite tired after all of that celebrating.

The last week of December, I got the chemotherapy that I had postponed. It wasn't too bad. We went to a friend's house on New Year's Eve for a few hours and watched one of the bowl games. Thanks for inviting us, Debbie! We came home to watch the ball drop on TV. Pretty exciting, aren't we?

Throughout the month of January, the kids went back to school. Ashley E. had the longest break (until almost the end of the month). It was so wonderful to have them at home and to have their friends visit us. I really miss them when they are at school.

My LAST chemotherapy treatment was January 6, 2015! I did not know that at the time, but I found out for sure when I saw the oncologist on January 27. I was very disappointed that we did not know so everyone could celebrate.

He had good news to report. My CT scan looked good; much of the cancer in my liver was converted to scar tissue, which means IT WAS KILLED OFF! There still is cancer in there, yet it is under control. This result is what Dr. L. was aiming for with the chemotherapy.

The end of treatment is a cause for celebration for many survivors of cancer. In some institutions, survivors ring a bell to signal to themselves and others that their treatment is over. This is not always a positive thing for many survivors (Liz is one of them), as they likely will receive additional treatment in the future or may still even have ongoing adjuvant treatment, such as hormone-blocking medications, which many women with breast cancer take for an extended period. So, ringing the bell may not mark the end of treatment but instead marks the passage from one phase to another. For women with metastatic disease, the aim is not to cure the cancer but to prolong survival and mitigate the symptoms associated with the spread of the cancer. This promotes quality of life (Reinert & Barrios, 2015).

I now am on a drug called fulvestrant. It is an estrogen antagonist that doesn't allow estrogen to bind with cancer cells. It is that binding that caused my cancer to grow. The drug is given intramuscularly in both cheeks of my buttocks! The liquid is very thick, so it has to be given as two shots. Damn, those suckers hurt! My butt was sore for about a week after those injections. I'm just impressed that the nurse found any muscle left back there!

I am getting the injections every two weeks right now to get the loading dose onboard. After that, I will have the shots once per month. I see the oncologist again at the end of February and will get another CT scan in the middle of April.

Fulvestrant is used for women with breast cancer that has spread and who were previously on other antihormonal medications, such as tamoxifen or an aromatase inhibitor. It generally is well tolerated, though some women have experienced gastrointestinal upset or joint pain or stiffness (Ishida et al., 2015).

Last weekend, my family surprised me with dinner at one of my favorite restaurants. My son and two of his friends (my adopted sons) were at the restaurant, which was a surprise for me. After we sat down, someone came up behind me and started to rub my shoulders. I turned around, and it was Ashley W.! I was so shocked because I never expected her to be home! She planned the whole thing and even made the reservations at the restaurant. She was home all weekend and drove back to Penn State on Monday morning. I ate dinner in shock, as I still couldn't believe they were able to surprise me like that! Ashley E. was not able to come home, but I did get to see her yesterday for a few hours. It was nice to celebrate the end of chemotherapy with my family. I received chemotherapy for almost eight months! Whew! Glad that part is over. I may have to have chemotherapy again at some point, so I am celebrating the end of this round and trying not to imagine what the future might hold.

I am working at least one day per week in the office and then doing some things at home. I am frustrated that I don't immediately feel better since stopping chemotherapy. I'm still so tired. Some days, my body feels like it's been hit by a truck. I understand that I have to be patient, but that is a hard thing for me to do. I just want my old self back!

The desire to be "normal" or "ordinary" and have one's old life back is universal among survivors of cancer, but it takes time and patience. As Liz readily admits, she finds it difficult to be patient!

Cancer-related fatigue is a frustrating experience with multiple contributing factors, including stress, medication side effects, lack of physical conditioning, pain, and sleep disturbances, among other treatment-related factors (Martz & Kirby, 2011). Feeling exhausted and like you were hit by a truck is a good description of cancer-related fatigue. One of the cardinal symptoms of this fatigue is that it is not really alleviated by rest or sleep and can persist for months or years after treatment is over.

Thank you again for all of your love, support, gifts, and prayers. Please keep praying for my continued healing, as this journey is not yet over. Maybe it is this dreary weather that makes me feel bad, despite the good news. I'm SO looking forward to spring.

March 14, 2015

One of my friends from work introduced me to Pack Health and their Cancer Pain and Fatigue program. Anyone can enroll for free in this program. You receive a box of goodies (OK, they call it a tool kit) in the mail that includes things like community resources, a caregiver guide, healthy eating guide, day tracker, and an exercise guide.

I had my first call today with my health advisor, Barb. For the next eight weeks, we will call each other every Thursday.

Pack Health (www.packhealth.com/cancer-facebook -support) is a for-profit business that provides some free services to people dealing with cancer and other chronic diseases. They also provide a "healthcare advisor" to help with lifestyle changes, education, and information about the specific disease for a nine-month period.

March 31, 2015

I hope you are starting to see some signs of spring where you are. We thought spring had started, only to have a covering of snow recently. However, it is supposed to be 70°F later this week in Pittsburgh. How crazy!

I am doing better. I saw my oncologist on March 24. He told me that everything looked good! I now am getting fulvestrant as an injection only once per month (down from two times per month). I'm sore for about a week and then OK for the rest of the month. I go back to see Dr. L. on April 21. I will have a CT scan early in the morning. He will have the results available that day. Good thing, because it is agonizing waiting to hear the results.

I'm still going to work one day a week, usually on Wednesdays. I have two conferences coming up in April about a week apart—a Health Information Management Systems Society (HIMSS) conference in Chicago and ONS Congress in Orlando.

I'm also walking at least three times per week. I have surpassed 10,000 steps over the past few days! I did not go today because of rain. I might melt in the rain (ha ha). The exercise does feel good; I'm hoping it will help me start to feel less tired, just as the evidence says!

Liz has been using her Fitbit®, a small electronic device that measures movement and steps taken, to motivate herself to exercise. Self-motivation has been shown to be effective in promoting physical activity. When this is accompanied by goal-setting, such as Liz's goal of 10,000 steps, it may be more effective (Tate, Lyons, & Valle, 2015). Liz feels good after exercising and is motivated to continue, as she hopes it will decrease her fatigue.

OK, gotta run. I submitted a book proposal, which was accepted, so I have to get moving on it. I already started it and plan to make Thursdays my writing day. It is easy to sit and write, as I can take a break when I get tired.

Talk to you soon. Keep those prayers and good wishes coming!

April 16, 2015

A lot has been happening over the last several weeks. I was having significant abdominal pain, knee pain, headaches, and shortness of breath. I chalked it up to side effects from the fulvestrant. However, the abdominal pain was pretty intense last week, so I talked with the nurse and the physician assistant (PA) at my oncologist's office. I then went into the office on April 10 and saw the PA, who examined me and could not find anything major. However, she was concerned with the increase in pain and the shortness of breath. I already had a CT scan scheduled for April 21, so they moved it up to April 15.

I was scheduled to attend the HIMSS conference from April 11 through April 16. Needless to say, I had to cancel my attendance. I was VERY disappointed yet did not want to go to a major conference feeling so bad. In addition, I was a nervous wreck about the CT scan showing something concerning. I received several emails and tweets from my pals who were really looking forward to seeing me. Oh well. I need to be sure nothing major is happening regarding my health.

I went to the office all day on Tuesday, April 14. It actually was a good day, as I kept busy thinking about work things and not the CT scan. I made sure I walked around to visit my staff and get in some exercise. I was slow going up and coming down the steps, but I made it!

I had the CT scan of my chest, abdomen, and pelvis on April 15. It was pretty anticlimactic. There were so many people in the waiting room. You have to sit there for an hour drinking the contrast fluid. As I looked around, I wondered who the patients were and who the caregivers were. It became more obvious when I saw some of them drink the same contrast fluid. Others had bald heads, so it was evident that those people were the patients. You just don't know what people are going through. Some may be at the end of their journey, while some might be newly diagnosed. I just kept praying for all of us.

I went home that day imagining all kinds of scenarios in my head. It was very difficult to think about anything else. I watched some TV and read a soap opera magazine to distract myself.

Waiting for test results is an agonizing process for many people. Focusing on the physical symptoms and worrying about what they might mean is a form of rumination or brooding, which is associated with anxiety and stress. Intrusive thoughts also are associated with stress. Some women may use avoidance (e.g., not adhering to treatment) to cope with stress (Soo & Sherman, 2015).

Mindfulness-based stress reduction (MBSR) has been shown to reduce distress and physical symptoms (Würtzen et al., 2015). MBSR began as a form of Buddhist meditation thousands of years ago. Jon Kabat-Zinn, the pioneer in this field in health care, has developed this therapy, which has been used in various disease states (Brotto & Goldmeier, 2015). Mindfulness practice is based on paying attention to something, such as an emotion, in the moment and with no judgment (Paulson, Davidson, Jha, & Kabat-Zinn, 2013). This might mean accepting worry and fear for what they are and not as things that are bad or negative. MBSR has been studied in women with breast cancer and has shown significant improvements in the occurrence of anxiety and depression (Gotink et al., 2015).

I did not sleep much last night, as I could not slow down my brain. It was very frustrating. At one point, I got on my phone under the covers (like I was 13!) and checked through Facebook—anything to think about something besides the results.

I called the oncologist's office early this morning and talked with Chris, the RN/nurse navigator. She has her OCN® (oncology certified nurse) certification and has been tremendous during this whole nightmare. She told me they had a very busy clinic day today and that Courtney (the PA) would look at my films (not really films but pictures on the computer) and call me when she had a chance. You know, that one simple phone call maybe lasted three minutes, but it was just what I needed to feel supported and not just another patient in a long line of phone calls to return.

Courtney called later in the afternoon and told me that the CT scan looked great! There was nothing in the chest and no additional cancer growth in my liver. She said there is a small amount of fluid (ascites) in my abdomen and pelvis, but it was not of major concern at this point. She said I will still see Dr. L. next Tuesday (April 21) and that we could discuss the other reasons for my pain.

I felt like a million dollars! Thank you, Lord, for the positive results! I have been praying night and day for God's support and His strength to help me continue my survivor course. I believe He has listened to me and has given me additional strength—not to mention a "great" CT scan.

Thanks for your thoughts and prayers. I will let you know how things go after I see the doctor on April 21.

May 2, 2015

We opened our pool today! What a grand sight to see that sparkling blue water. I always feel fabulous when we open the pool. It signifies the beginning of summer to me, even though it is still spring. I know I can't lie in the sun to get a tan and will be especially careful when I am outside.

Avoiding sun damage by wearing sunscreen and not deliberately tanning is an important preventive measure for survivors of cancer. Sun exposure also can cause problems for people on anticancer medications; survivors should be told this when prescribed those medications. However, vitamin D is important, particularly for women on endocrine-blocking medications. The sun is a good source of vitamin D. Some survivors limit their exposure to the sun to just 10 minutes a day to encourage the body's own vitamin D stores, while others choose to take vitamin D supplements in addition to calcium.

May 7, 2015

I am sad today, as I would have been married to my previous husband for 32 years. He has been gone for 12 years now. R.I.P. Pat. Our children are graduating from college this year, and I will be there! We will miss you.

I also finished my Pack Health program. My advisor and I reviewed all that I had accomplished in eight weeks. Much of the information I already knew, but it was a nice review. The exercise information helped me the most. I knew that exercise was important to my recovery, but I just couldn't get going with it. I guess I was too lazy. However, I did not want to admit to Barb (my advisor) that I still wasn't doing anything each week. Therefore, as the weather got nicer, I started walking around the neighborhood. I started out slow and worked up to 3.46 miles and more than 10,000 steps per day! I used my Fitbit to keep track of everything and made it to an 18-minute mile. It doesn't sound like much, but it was great progress for me! I now try to walk at least three times per week or every day if the weather cooperates.

Liz is motivated to be physically active and has been walking, but there also is a degree of social desirability in her persistence with exercising. She did not want to appear to be failing the recommended exercise routine provided by her health advisor. Having a healthcare provider involved in her care supports the evidence that these individuals motivate, encourage, and provide information that promotes adherence to an exercise regimen (Blaney et al., 2010). This accountability to others also can occur when one exercises as part of a social group (McArthur, Dumas, Woodend, Beach, & Stacey, 2014). A supervised exercise program has been shown to have benefits to motivation as many as five years after the activity started (Trinh, Mutrie, Campbell, Crawford, & Courneya, 2014).

May 14, 2015

Since I have started walking, I have noticed that my stamina has improved. I just worked two days in a row and did not fall asleep in any meetings. That's another milestone for me. Two days AND no sleeping in the afternoon; these results motivate me to keep walking. Thank you, Lord, for getting through to me. I am still tired in the evening, yet it is such a terrific life improvement for me. I'm also getting to know more of the neighbors and their dogs. God is good!

May 21, 2015

I worked two days this week and actually feel OK. I can feel myself getting tired in the afternoon. My colleague continues to be my chauffeur both to and from work. I am so grateful for her help. I don't feel comfortable driving at this time, and she has made it possible for me to go back to work.

Today also was the Kenny Chesney concert. I attend his concerts every time he comes to Pittsburgh. I took a nap in the afternoon so I would have enough energy to get through the evening. I even drove home because my daughter had been drinking. (Don't worry, she is old enough—almost 23!)

Balancing activity and rest is an important strategy to manage cancer-related fatigue. Liz is doing everything she is supposed to in order to improve her stamina; she is exercising, asking for help with daily activities (e.g., driving to and from work), and resting when she can. A graduated return to work also is important to her success. Not every workplace will make these accommodations. Some people have to resign from their jobs because they cannot meet the demands of their job duties.

June 8, 2015

I drove to work for the very first time since the little fender bender I had several months ago. I had been "nursing" a very swollen belly. In fact, it felt like I was six months pregnant. My abdomen was very tight, so I called the nurse navigator at my oncologist's office. She told me to go to the ED. Well, I have ascites, and they found cancer cells in that fluid. The docs did a paracentesis and put me back in the hospital.

June 10, 2015

I had a pretty good day today, resting and enjoying the pain meds. I was very comfortable. Around 8:30 pm, I got up to go to the bathroom, dragging my IV pole and PleurX (the drainage system for my ascites) with me. On the way back to bed, I stopped to look at some magazines on a chair. All of a sudden, I could feel myself losing control of my body. I have never felt like that before. Then, I fell to the floor with the IVs and PleurX. I tried to catch myself, but the sheets on the bed just pulled out. I assessed myself (trauma nurse till the end) and could not find any injuries. I was not anywhere near the call light, so I yelled for help.

One of the nurses came in and asked me if I was OK, as I was lying on the floor. No trauma survey by her! I could have busted my head open and still said I was OK. Luckily, I didn't. I was so embarrassed and kept apologizing: "I know this fall is screwing up your June numbers. I'm so sorry."

Each unit has to report the number of falls and what happened to the Joint Commission. I felt like such a klutz.

The nurse helped me get situated and back to bed. There was no damage to the IV or the PleurX. She put my bed on alarm and told me to call the nurse if I needed something. No more getting out of bed by myself. Of course, I had to see if it really worked. I stood up from the bed and the alarm went off.

Oh yeah, it worked.

A nurse came rushing in. I apologized and said I had dropped something on the floor. What a trip!

June 11, 2015

Happy birthday, Amanda Panda! She would have been 28 years old today. I hope she is celebrating in heaven with her dad.

June 12, 2015

An abdominal drain was implanted in the left upper quadrant of my abdomen. The tubing is connected directly to a PleurX so that it drains continuously. It was draining about 2,000 cc (to start) from my peritoneum. I'm now down to about 150 cc draining every other day. Thanks for caring about me. It's been rough!

The development of ascites (fluid in the abdominal cavity) is not a good sign, as Liz acknowledges (Eichbaum et al., 2006). Treatment starts with draining the fluid to make the patient more comfortable. A drain may be left in so that the patient does not have to have a needle inserted. This also allows the fluid to drain continually, enabling the patient to be more comfortable, as fluid does not build up.

June 14, 2015

I had an emotional meltdown today. I thought there was a hematoma around my drainage tube. A doctor from internal medicine (essentially, the guy on call) came in and examined my belly. I *insisted* that I could feel a blood clot and wanted one of my oncologists. After some convincing on the doctor's part, I calmed down. The doctor and my husband thought this reaction was because of changes in my medicine, specifically a new narcotic for pain.

June 15, 2015

Somehow, they started me on new medication without my knowledge. I was extremely pissed! I mentioned it to the day shift nurse, but she was finishing her shift. I don't think my concerns went anywhere. The evening shift nurse was very busy, and I barely saw her. The night shift nurse was shocked that no one had taken the time to explain the drugs. For instance, I had never heard of the drug Opana® (oxymorphone hydrochloride) and had no idea it was a narcotic pain med!

I also discovered that the cap to the port in my chest was missing. I immediately let the nurse know, as I was afraid I would get an infection, then sepsis, and then die. I tend to think of the worst scenarios. The nurse had no idea that it was gone, so she scrubbed it vigorously and put on a new sterile cap.

June 16, 2015

I was discharged from the hospital today. Here is a list of my questions before I left. Some were answered by the physician, and some were answered by the nurse.

- How often do I see Dr. L. in the office?
- How long do I need to be on capecitabine?
- You want the fulvestrant stopped, right?
- How often do I get my blood drawn and tested?
- How often should I drain my peritoneum? What is the cutoff number for the amount of drainage each time? (I was told that my port needs to be flushed with heparin at least every four weeks.)
- How does this all affect my prognosis?

June 19, 2015

I met Cari today. She is the home health nurse who will be helping me manage everything at home. I was nervous going home—can you believe a nurse is afraid? There just were so many things going on with meds, drainage tubes, nausea and vomiting, pain management, etc.

Cari drained 250 cc of straw-colored fluid from my belly and explained everything she did. She examined the tube insertion site, as I was worried about infection. It was fine. She will check this each time she removes the dressing. She was very caring, and I could tell she was good at her job.

June 21, 2015

So much for the first day of summer! My blood pressure was very low, and I ended up being admitted to the hospital through the ED. They thought I was dehydrated and that I might have an infection. The nurse drained about 60 cc from my tube and sent it to the laboratory to check for infection. She saw my belly was still bloated, so she drained another 600 cc. They also stopped the capecitabine because of the possible infection.

June 24, 2015

I was discharged from the hospital today. Before I left, they weighed me. I was 156 pounds—that's a lot for me. I had a ton of fluid in my peritoneum. I'm not sure why one of the nurses didn't drain me before I went home.

June 25, 2015

I went for my first haircut today! It still feels so wonderful to have hair. Lots of curls are coming in, so it just needed "shaped up." Darcie also covered up the gray, as a lot of gray hair came through.

July 1, 2015

Happy birthday to my mom. She would have been 83 today. She died three years ago. I miss her so much. With all of this medical stuff going on, I just want to sit on her lap and have her tell me it will all be OK.

July 2, 2015

One of my home health nurses came today and disagreed with some of the things the previous nurse (not Cari) did. We were caught in the middle and didn't know what to do. She ended up examining me and not draining anything. It was weird.

It's so difficult seeing so many different people with different ways of doing things. As I said, we really are caught in the middle.

July 3, 2015

The home health nurse for today was Jennifer. She was much nicer and drained 410 cc of yellow fluid. I'm down to 135 pounds.

July 4, 2015

It was rather quiet today, which was a HUGE improvement from last year when I was in the hospital on July 4! We had family over, the kids swam in the pool, and the hubby made dinner on the grill. I sat outside under an umbrella to stay out of the sun.

July 6, 2015

Cari was here today. She drained 450 cc of amber fluid. She also examined me and was looking for side effects from the medicine. It was so great to see her. I hope we can arrange for her to be my permanent nurse.

July 8, 2015

The home health nurse was here today and drained 100 cc of amber fluid. My examination was fine.

I also went to lunch with a dear friend of mine, Felicia, who also is a survivor of breast cancer. She did the driving! When we got to the restaurant, I felt so nauseated I ended up vomiting at the end of the parking lot. I hate the nausea and vomiting! We had lunch (soup for me) and headed home. On the way, we had to pull over to the side of the road so I could throw up again. Very embarrassing! Felicia was wonderful and handed me some tissues.

July 10, 2015

I saw Dr. L. today and started a new routine. I will be on capecitabine for one week and then off of it for a week. So, I will have a week to recover from the side effects.

July 30, 2015

I spent the rest of the month wrestling with constipation and diarrhea. It was awful, and I will definitely spare you the details. We tried different meds, combinations of meds, etc. It was a very rough road. Cari continued to see me throughout the month. She really helped me get through this mess.

July 31, 2015

HAPPY BIRTHDAY TO ME! I made it to 59 years. Whew! One of my goals has been met. Now I have to change it and hope to get to 60. I will expect a big party, so you all better start planning now!

I had an appointment with Dr. L. today. I took in cupcakes for both of our birthdays (his is July 22). I walked around to visit nurses, staff, and everyone else I interact with to thank them for working so hard. I saved two cupcakes for Dr. L. and gave one to Chris, his nurse navigator. She was so surprised. It felt really good to reward everyone with something as a small thank-you for keeping me alive. What a great feeling!

On a sad note: We discussed the schedule for the capecitabine. I was under the impression that I would take it a while and then be done—just like the IV chemotherapy. Instead, Dr. L. told me that the goal is to keep the cancer inactive, which is what the drug is doing. So, I will need to be on some type of oral chemotherapy for the rest of my life. I was so shocked, and it took a while to sink in. Yes, I cried. I thought there was an end to this nightmare. When I got home, I just lay in bed and cried. Ashley W. and my Aunt Gail cried with me and did their best to comfort me.

August 3, 2015

August was a relatively quiet month. I kept up with my meds, Cari continued to see me several times per week, and I saw Dr. L. every two weeks. I also got some exercise by walking. In fact, I was up to five miles at 18 minutes per mile at one point. It doesn't sound like very much, but for me, it felt like a miracle. I never walked when I was healthy. Now, I really enjoy it.

On my walks, I go through the neighborhoods and listen to music. I love when it is warm and there is a big blue sky. It really helps my mental health. I'm not looking forward to the cold weather and snow. No walking outside for me in the freezing cold!

September 2, 2015

Today was Ashley W.'s birthday. She turned 23 today. It also is a very important day for me personally, as I was officially diagnosed with breast cancer on this date in 2009. As you may recall, I waited a few days to tell my children. It was so hard to keep such important information from my family, although I did tell my husband. They all weren't too worried because they believed that the surgeon (Dr. M.) would just cut out the cancer and it would be gone. I was not quite that accepting, as I learned about the lumpectomy, radiation therapy, etc.

It has now been six years since I was officially diagnosed. I was cancer-free for ALMOST five years. In fact, I kind of started feeling like this whole process was done. I really thought that if I made it to five years, I was cured.

September 3, 2015

I had another CT scan today just to see where things are at this point.

Labor Day weekend, 2015

I had a good weekend chilling with friends and family. I love having a pool so people can come and enjoy it with us!

September 4 was the last day taking capecitabine for this week. I am off for a week and then back on it next Friday. I do my best to enjoy the days I am off of it. Unfortunately, the side effects show up during that week off. It feels like a holiday to me when I complete the week on the drug. I get so happy that I don't have to take it for another week. I tried to talk my oncologist into one week on and two weeks off. He didn't buy it and feels the schedule he has for me right now is the best one to keep the cancer from growing. That rationale was fine with me, so one off and one on will continue.

This is a good example of two things:

1. Liz recognizes that she feels better when she is off her anticancer medication. However, with the schedule she is on, Liz hardly has time to recover in the week off before she has to start taking it again. While her blood counts may improve in the week that she does not take the medication, she still feels unwell.

2. Liz is trying to negotiate a different schedule for the medication so that her quality of life improves, but her oncologist has to balance her quality of life and keeping the cancer under control. Even though Liz does not get what she wants, she is listened to and an explanation is given. This is a good example of the person-centered care described earlier.

September 8, 2015

Today is my eighth wedding anniversary. I feel bad that I could not go out and get a nice gift for my husband. I didn't even have a card for him, and I am such a card freak. I love giving them and getting them. He, of course, gave me a beautiful card, body butter, and chocolate-covered strawberries. Yum! Wonder what the body butter is for?

September 9, 2015

I am so sick of all these medications I am taking! The co-pays are horrendous, and for many of them, we need a new prescription because they are only good for one time. One example is oxymorphone. It is a schedule II narcotic, so I understand why they do not refill it. Other drugs are not as simple. They are not narcotics, so I don't understand why they are labeled "No Refills."

> While some medications cannot be prescribed with refills, others can (e.g., antinausea medication). Requiring the patient to get additional or repeat prescriptions means that the patient has to make an appointment, go to the doctor's office, wait in the waiting room, etc. All of this takes time away from home, is tiring, and potentially exposes the patient to germs and viruses in the doctor's office. This could be dealt with so much better. However, another side to this problem exists. Often, patients continue taking medication that they may not need if they have refills prescribed. Having to see the oncologist regularly allows for an assessment of how patients are feeling and a review of the medications they are taking (allowing potential adjustments to these medications according to current health status).

Thank goodness the pharmacy we use has been terrific. We know the pharmacists and the pharmacy technician by name and vice versa. They frequently call us to review something about a medicine or to say that they have not heard back from a doctor for authorization. At times, they call the doctor's office directly if they have a specific question. I usually call the nurse navigator (Chris) for Dr. L. She takes care of the rest. I feel very much at ease once Chris is involved. There is a level of trust I have with her.

There was one time not too long ago that I was completely out of a certain drug that I really needed (can't remember which one—thank you, chemo brain). I suggested that the pharmacy give us five to hold me over until the actual prescription had been reauthorized. Because they knew us as "frequent flyers," they were fine with giving me just a few of those pills until the full refill was available. They knew that we were not selling pills on the streets!

September 10, 2015

I went back to work today. I provided my release to return to work so that everything was legal. My colleague offered to drive me to the office, as I am not really driving too much yet. Our offices are currently being renovated, so there were people working in different places, and some areas were closed on the first and second floors of the building. It was crazy! I had to go around and find my coworkers. I finally found them in a temporary place. What fun playing hide-and-seek! It also was good exercise.

I was completely exhausted when I got home. I took a nap to get some of my energy back.

September 11, 2015

My daughter and I went to see Jason Aldean at a large concert pavilion west of the city. I signed up for his fan club and got to buy tickets way before others. I love going to concerts and love to sing along to the songs with the artist. I missed Jason last year because I was too sick to go. I gave my ticket to my daughter, and she took a friend. This time, I even drove to and from the venue. I was psyched from the concert and singing his songs on the way home. I had no problem staying awake.

September 14, 2015

The visiting nurse, Cari, has been seeing me at home two or three times per week to check on my overall status and drain the peritoneal fluid through the rubber tubing in the left lower quadrant of my abdomen. She also cleans around the tubing insertion site, as well as the larger area where the dressing is placed. At first, it was really awkward. That feeling changed to trust (there's that "T" word again) as we got to know one another. She also has a good relationship with Chris, Dr. L.'s nurse navigator. I can ask Cari any question, and she'll either give me an answer or check another source and get right back to me. I never feel like she is rushing to get to the rest of her patients.

Trust is an important component of the nurse–patient relationship and is seen as a component of a shared covenant (promise or commitment) between the nurse and patient (Coffey, 2006). Trust is established when the nurse meets a need for the patient, is respectful, pays attention to the time spent with the patient, and provides continuity of care (Leslie & Lonneman, 2016). Patients tend to have a general trust of nurses. This is based on specific actions by the nurse, including professional competence and caring, good communication skills, empathy, and being worthy of the trust placed on them (Dinc & Gastmans, 2013). Trust can be broken, usually because the nurse shows a lack of respect for the patient, incompetent care, or unethical behaviors (Leslie & Lonneman, 2016).

Allowing a home health nurse into one's home adds another layer to the nurse–patient relationship. At first, the nurse is a guest in the patient's home and must act accordingly. As the relationship builds over time, the location of care means that the relationship can be deeper and more intimate. There is a need for reciprocity in this relationship. Over time, the nurse can become almost a friend with a mutual sharing of ideas and trust (Wälivaara, Sävenstedt, & Axelsson, 2013).

There were a few times when Cari would be off or on vacation and another person would have to see me. One time, it was a male.

That was awkward for me, yet I made it through his examination and drainage. Another time, a very nice older woman came. I felt more at ease with her. Maybe it was the male/female thing, as I was less concerned when my nurse was female. Oh well, this happened only a few times.

This is a good example of some of the challenges of home health nursing. When a stand-in nurse has to visit Liz, the trust is not there. Without this trust, there can be awkwardness and even a lack of comfort. In these instances, any relationship between nurse and patient will be more superficial (Wälivaara et al., 2013).

September 24, 2015

Saw Dr. L. today. He said the numbers (blood work) were good and that he was very pleased with my progress. I told him about my book and that he would be in it. He just laughed. I also told him the two of us will be doing a presentation together. He asked, "When?" I explained that it will be sometime in the future as I get better. He laughed again.

I feel like we have an interesting relationship. When he comes into the room, the first thing he says is, "Your scan is great!" He is so in touch with his patients that he knows that we sit there in fear waiting for the results. He even told me that he purposely says that first to put the patients at ease. That is very important to me.

He can be very stern, and I can argue right back with him. I have cried multiple times in front of him and also have said the "F" word (just once) in front of him. I value his medical knowledge and his affection for me. When the testing is good, he gives me a big hug. If there are serious things to discuss, he sits down in a chair, pulls it over, and talks to me at my level, instead of just hovering over me.

He answers my questions, and my husband's, my son's, my daughters', and my Aunt Gail's (when she is in town). He asks, "What do you think about that?" or "What would you like to talk about?" He is very passionate about safe care and will explain things straight to me, even though I may not want to hear them. If I start to cry, he pauses for a minute and then asks, "What do you want to talk about?" or "What are you afraid of?" I always tell him that I am afraid to die and leave my children. That fear has not changed one bit. I think about it a lot.

Liz clearly appreciates the time that her oncologist spends talking with her and her family and answering all of their questions. Patients are sensitive to a physician's responses to their emotional cues. When the physician recognizes that the patient is feeling something, even if the patient doesn't say it out loud or show an emotional response, the identification of the emotional cue and the invitation to discuss what is upsetting the patient leads to patient satisfaction (Blanch-Hartigan, 2013).

At one point, I was confused about the chemotherapy. I thought after I finished a few rounds of capecitabine that I would be done. It was kind of like the first time with radiation. When I was done, I would go back to my regular life. Dr. L. reminded me that I could be on chemotherapy for the rest of my life. I started to cry, as I saw no relief in the future. I was incredibly sad and did not see a future for me if I always had to be on chemotherapy. It was difficult for me to change my thinking, but he gave me all the time I needed to readjust. My sister and husband were in the room with me.

I have such respect for this physician and trust him with my life. He asks my opinion on things yet helps me understand when there are no other options. My first oncologist, Dr. O., gave me two years to live when I saw her in June 2014. I am determined to live longer than that. Dr. L. is being aggressive with my treatment to give me the best chance at survival.

How a physician communicates with a patient is the basis of trust in the relationship (Kowalski et al., 2009). The ability of the physician to assess the unmet needs of a patient is important in providing the supportive care and information that the patient needs (Lelorain et al., 2015). As much as she admires and trusts her physician, there was a breakdown in communication about the length of time that she would be taking the capecitabine, a medication that significantly affects her quality of life.

Liz initially did not understand something about her treatment—that she would be on it forever. She may have been told this at one point, but the information was not retained. She could have been told this information in a way she did not understand, at a time that she could not take it in, or while she was distressed (when information often is not heard or remembered). Or, because she is a nurse, it may have been assumed that she understood everything about her treatment. But she is a patient and a woman with cancer. Assumptions cannot be made that detract from her basic need for information about her treatment. She has had multiple interactions with her oncologist and other members of the healthcare team who should have been assessing her understanding of the treatment regimen, including the length of time that she will be taking her medications (Brédart et al., 2013).

New medications offer the hope of extending life for those living with metastatic disease, something described as "chronic metastatic disease." Individuals who are part of this new and unique group of survivors describe their experience as one of unpredictability and without a road map (Thorne et al., 2013).

For a while, I was determined to get more information about live-donor liver transplants. I talked with friends and physicians I knew. I thought for sure they could cut out the cancer and give me a piece of a healthy donor liver. Well, Dr. L. must have gotten tired of me asking him about it all the time. He finally told me that the last thing I needed was immunosuppression, which was necessary with a transplant. Once my body became as immune suppressed as possible, as required by the transplanted organ to decrease the potential for rejection, it also would allow the cancer to grow. I never thought of it that way. I wished he would have explained this a while ago so I wasn't nagging him all the time!

Oncologists are seen by women as a primary source of information (Lewis, Yee, Kilbreath, & Willis, 2015). Once Liz's oncologist explained the reason why a liver transplant could not be considered, the rationale was clear. However, it appears that she had asked about it before and had thought that it was possible. So, why were opportunities missed in the past to explain this to her?

September 25, 2015

Patrick, Ashley W., and I went to Buffalo for the weekend. The daughter of dear friends of ours was getting married. We ate dinner at the hotel and saw some of the wedding party at the bar. We all had a great time talking with them and meeting new people.

September 26, 2015

The wedding was beautiful! I cried because the bride looked so beautiful. We knew this family before their kids were even born. We met them on our honeymoon in 1983 at a resort in Jamaica. When Pat died, the entire family came to Pittsburgh for the viewing and funeral.

I don't know if I will live long enough to see my kids get married. That feeling comes deep from my soul and causes me intense grief. I don't want to cheat my kids out of a grandmother or cheat myself out of having grandchildren and fussing over them. However, only my son has a steady girlfriend, so I'm not seeing weddings or babies for quite a while. That worries me. Also, watching the father/daughter dance usually brings me to tears, as my daughter will never have that. Her dad will not walk her down the aisle. Her brother will do it, but it won't be the same. If I am not there, those poor kids will have unimaginable pain.

> Here, Liz describes the existential suffering that so many women with metastatic cancer endure. In the midst of a celebration, she sees what she will lose with an early death—the opportunity to see her children married, to watch them have children of their own, and her own dreams of being a grandmother. It also brings to the forefront the memory and pain of the loss of her second husband.

There were several hours between the wedding and the reception, so we drove over to Niagara Falls. My kids did not remember camping up there when they were little. It was a beautiful, warm, sunny day. The only thing that hurt were my feet from all the walking I did in high heels. I finally took them off and carried them back to the car. Ashley W. was having the same problem, and her heels were much higher than mine. We were both running around in bare feet!

The reception was so much fun. It was great that we could laugh and enjoy the music. The cancer feeling went away for a while! There was a live band that was really great. I even danced for the first time with my son—fast and slow. I didn't realize that he was so talented.

It was so fun with just the three of us, and I kept thanking God for this time with them. All of these people were coming up to me and telling me how great I looked. That was nice.

I was pretty tired and went back to the hotel by shuttle around 10:30 pm. I really hated to cut out early but was trying to listen to my body. My kids were worried about me leaving early by myself. I assured them that I could get back on my own. My son is very protective of me and always checks to see what I need. I love his concern for me. I got back to our room, climbed under the covers, and watched TV. Of course, I fell asleep. The kids got back to the room around 3 am. They had so much fun.

September 27, 2015

After we checked out of the hotel, we went over to the family's house to continue the celebration. We were not drinking because my son had to drive us home, which is about a four-hour drive. It was fun to see everyone and talk about the wedding. They had some really funny stories.

I am talking so much about this weekend because I got to spend quality time with my son and daughter. It's not often that we are all together, and I wanted to just breathe in their love. I really needed some time when I didn't think of cancer every hour of the day. This weekend provided that much-needed time to just live my life. I still had pain and took my meds, but I had other things to talk about besides cancer, which was a wonderful break.

September 30, 2015

The skin around the tube's insertion site is red. I thought it was cellulitis. There was clearly some type of infection. I took pictures of it and sent them to Cari and Dr. L.'s office. The diagnosis was cellulitis. Chris called in a prescription for an antibiotic to clear it up.

I was really nervous about the infection and worried about how bad it could get. I had seen really gross wounds in my days as a clinical nurse and knew I did not want any type of major wound on MY body. Yuck! I also was worried about getting sepsis if this cellulitis didn't clear up. I was worried over nothing. I took the medicine every day and it cleared up very nicely.

October 2, 2015

I spent the day researching options for financial assistance. As I mentioned before, the costs and co-payments are ridiculous. We are not eligible for some grants because our combined salaries are too high. That still does not justify $2,500 for a drug! Rumor has it that capecitabine is going generic. That may make the cost a bit more realistic for this drug.

The cost of anticancer medications is a source of distress to patients, their families, and increasingly to the oncology medical community. Medical expenses pose a significant economic burden on survivors of cancer, both soon after diagnosis and in the years after treatment (Guy et al., 2013). This economic burden is experienced most commonly in adults younger than the age of 64 and includes a psychological component, as survivors worry about their financial status and stability (Yabroff et al., 2015). When new medications are used, an increased risk of side effects often exists. This also increases the costs of care (Niraula et al., 2014). The increased financial burden of the costs of cancer care affects quality of life for survivors (Fenn et al., 2014). Some survivors may neglect their medical care because of financial hardships (Kent et al., 2013).

The high costs of cancer are the result of a number of factors, including the pharmaceutical companies who manufacture the drugs and pass the costs of research, development, and marketing to the patient; healthcare providers who prescribe medications that are expensive; and the insurance industry, which also passes these increasing costs of treatment to the patient—the most vulnerable link in this chain (Meropol et al., 2009).

When a drug loses patent protection and can be manufactured by companies that make generic versions, the prices often go down and the medication becomes more affordable, lessening the financial burden for the patient.

October 15, 2015

I rode to work with a colleague. She is so very helpful—I could not work if I didn't have a ride. Sometimes, she even gets me a chocolate chip muffin from one of the coffee places. It always is such a treat. I'm going to get her something nice for helping me.

This ride was a bit different than our usual commute. I forgot to take my ondansetron this morning. You can probably see where this is going! On the way to work on a major expressway, I had to stop. My colleague pulled over as fast as she could without getting hit by someone else. I jumped out of the car, leaned on a guardrail, and threw up. I was so embarrassed, but I felt a little better. My colleague felt really bad, as if she was driving wrong. I told her it was because I forgot to take the ondansetron before I left the house. I did not have any meds with me and was nauseated all day. What an awful feeling! I held up till 2:30 pm, then we left to go home. I took an ondansetron as soon as I got home and went to bed.

This is one area that really frustrates me. Just when I think I'm getting better, yet another issue strikes. I don't like to cause a scene.

I appreciate that everybody is trying to help. I just want to fit back into the corporation. I HATE having to need other people to help me with mundane tasks. For example, I cannot open the lid off a jar. I have to go to someone else to get the lid off for me. My fingers are not strong enough. I'm also experiencing dizziness, where I am afraid I will fall. I lean onto anyone's arm, hand, etc., to keep me stable. My proprioception and the general dexterity of my hands are terrible now. I'm blaming it on chemotherapy and not my age. I'm still young at 59, don't you think?

The activity restrictions that Liz refers to are called long-term or late effects of treatment. They may persist for years after treatment (long-term effects) or are symptoms that occur long after treatment is over (late effects). One of the side effects of Liz's chemotherapy is problems with the nerves affecting the hands and feet. Patients often complain of numbness and tingling, which can affect walking. They may fall or are not sure of their footing and are afraid of falling. This also may affect hand strength, as Liz described. There's also a suggestion that surgery to the breast can result in numbness in the arm on the side of the affected breast (Tasmuth, von Smitten, & Kalso, 1996).

October 18, 2015

I found enough energy to go to the Steelers game today. We have season tickets, and I usually am obsessive about going to every home game. I missed several last year when I was on chemotherapy and also have missed several home games this year. We sold most of our tickets to help recoup our investment. It was windy and very cold. I must face that I just don't have the same stamina, as we left early and went to my sister's house for dinner. By the end of dinner, I was falling asleep.

October 21, 2015

Today was Think Pink Day at ONS. I started this effort in 2011, when I began working there in April of that year. Anyone who wants to participate decorates their area and wears pink for the day—even the guys! We then take a picture of everyone together and post it in our dining room for all of the office staff, guests, board members, etc., to see. It is so exciting for me to see more and more people participating in the office. We have several survivors of breast cancer on our staff and are dedicated to seeing things get better for this group. It is such a blessing to see so many people in pink and to celebrate with the other survivors in our company.

November 1, 2015

Went to another Steelers game today. I run out of energy pretty quickly, so we did not stay till the end. I used to be the one who said we would never leave early, no matter how much we were winning or losing. Oh well, that feeling changed when I was diagnosed with metastatic cancer. The diagnosis put my life on a new trajectory.

Living with metastatic disease has been described as "living under the shadow of death" (Sarenmalm et al., 2009) and requires adjustment in all aspects of life. Everything changes—life itself is uncertain, the prognosis is unknown, and changes occur in role functioning and relationships (Krigel, Myers, Befort, Krebill, & Klemp, 2014). Women with metastatic disease describe that their life becomes medicalized and that they are less active because of symptoms such as fatigue and pain (Vilhauer, 2008). Liz remarks on this in her entry about leaving a football game early, something she would not have done before she was diagnosed with metastatic cancer.

November 3, 2015

My sister is getting married on May 14, 2016. She's asked me to be her matron of honor! We were out shopping for dresses tonight. We both found one. She asked the girls to be junior bridesmaids and Patrick to be a big boy ring bearer.

It was so fun, although I was still thinking: *Will I be here for her wedding?* That's almost the two-year deadline for my life, as per my first oncologist. I keep coming up with these milestones, such as:

- I want to be alive for my sister's wedding.
- I want to see my children get married.
- I want to see my children have children.
- I just want more time to do the things I procrastinated!
- I WANT MORE TIME!

Planning for the future almost is impossible for those living with metastatic disease. Liz succinctly and poignantly shares her wishes for her future. They center on the loving relationships she has with family and the existential distress related to having limited time.

Despite the fun Liz had picking out a dress for her sister's wedding, nagging doubts crept into her mind, all focused on the reality of an early death and its influence on her family (Mosher et al., 2013).

November 9, 2015

Today always is a sad day for me. My daughter Amanda was pronounced brain dead at the hospital where she had surgery 14 years ago. It was awful when we had to tell her brother and sister. Friends picked them up and brought them to the hospital. I think about Amanda a lot and hope her last minutes of life were peaceful. I don't think so, with them jamming that nasogastric tube down her throat. We never did find out what really happened. There definitely was a "code of silence" at this hospital, and it was NOT a children's hospital. See her website at www.panda-llc.com.

November 22, 2015

I still have those darn mouth sores, or mucositis, as folks like to call it. I am using a special mouth rinse that has helped enormously. It is ridiculously expensive yet does the trick. I tried using a coupon, but the manufacturer would not accept it. I had to purchase it directly from them. Let's hope it gets more widespread use so the price comes down!

November 26, 2015
Thanksgiving

Today was Thanksgiving, and it was our turn to make dinner. We go to my sister's house for Christmas.

My Aunt Gail came in from Canada to be with us. She helped with some things, but it was my husband who did most of the cooking. It was a fabulous meal; I think everyone enjoyed it. It got pretty quiet as we were all stuffing our faces! The kids cleaned up while the rest of us sat around the table talking about lots of things. It was wonderful that people did not just run off after dinner.

The image of Liz's family sitting around the table and eating a traditional and delicious Thanksgiving meal almost is like a Rockwell painting. Liz is trying hard to maintain a sense of normality by participating in regular social occasions, despite not being able to do what she would usually do; her husband cooked most of the meal and her aunt helped. This is one strategy that women living with metastatic disease use to live well under the constraints of the disease—maintaining normality while reevaluating what is important and doing what they can do while letting go of what they cannot (Lewis, Willis, Yee, & Kilbreath, 2016).

Of course, I thought about how this could be my last Thanksgiving with my family. After everyone left, I went and looked at some old photos of Thanksgiving when the kids were young and Pat and Amanda were with us. It was neat to see how different we look today. During those earlier years, we didn't think about death and dying. Those were very innocent times. I miss them.

Yet reality creeps in, making Liz aware of the shadow that her illness has brought into their lives. She mourns what she had and what has been lost.

December 2, 2015

I had a CT scan in the morning and saw Dr. L. in the afternoon. During that lag time between appointments, we went to a diner in the area to eat lunch. Again, Dr. L. walked into the room and first told me my CT was great! He was very pleased. Of course, I hugged him.

My son, daughter, sister, and husband all were there. Dr. L. took the time to answer all of our questions. I love this guy. He said I don't have to come back for six weeks! It is the first time I will not be seen over such a long period. I can always call the office if I need something.

At last, Liz receives some good news! However, tempered with the good news is a small nagging fear about not being seen as often by her oncologist.

December 10, 2015

Today is the 12th anniversary of Pat's death. I kept replaying the details from that night over and over in my head. Telling my children that their father had died was the most heartbreaking thing I have ever done. We all cried so hard. Things were so up in the air that we didn't know what the next steps would be. I decided that I had to wait until Ashley was a bit more stable and in less pain before telling her about her father. I felt that telling her right away might take away her will to live. She and her dad were close. She talked to me later and couldn't understand why this happened to her dad, yet she still was alive. She was in so much physical and emotional pain that I did not want to add to her grief. The crash happened on a Wednesday. We told Ashley about her dad on Sunday.

This day has become even more important to me since being diagnosed with metastatic breast cancer. I want to support my kids and remind them of the wonderful things we've been able to do. I want to do as much as possible for them and with them in case I die before the holidays in 2016. Unfortunately, my cancer shortens this equation and takes away even more time, considering we are constantly fighting with our insurers to cover some of the more expensive treatments.

Reflections

I used to tell my kids that it was so great that my parents, brother, and sister all were still alive. Not many people can say that their primary family unit is still all together. Amanda's and Pat's deaths sure helped us wake up to see how fragile life and family really are. We lived our adjusted lives with just Patrick, Ashley, and me. It took us a while to get used to functioning as a family of three.

When I was first diagnosed in September 2009, it was hard for me to realize that cancer was growing in my right breast (Thelma, remember?). I did not feel anything and was shocked when the doctor told me about those tiny calcifications. I was lucky that it was found early and that my treatment did not include chemotherapy.

When the cancer came back in my entire liver, I was so upset. I thought the drugs I was taking were supposed to keep it from returning. I did not once associate my abdominal pain with metastasis to my liver or anywhere else in my body.

I was working full time at a job I loved, including all of the opportunities it provided. One of my areas of responsibility was publications, and I received a copy of every book we published. These books are wonderful and taught me a lot about oncology. In fact, we were setting up a visit to our cancer center to help me learn more about oncology nursing right before my diagnosis. I didn't really know much about oncology nursing, even though I had been a nurse for around 30 years. I just couldn't believe this cancer thing was happening to me! I was happy, healthy (I thought), and living the dream with my family. All three kids were in college, which definitely hurt our budget, but I was so excited that they were on their way to college degrees. I had a good marriage, my loving husband had a good job, and I was enjoying my blended family.

The relapse in May 2014 was quite a shock to me. I had been living a good life, was approaching the five-year magic number for survivors of cancer, and thought I would be "cured." That was not to be.

The next two years were brutal with the IV chemotherapy, all of its side effects, and the multiple hospital admissions. I sure learned a lot and told many of my caregivers that I was writing a book about my experiences as a nurse-turned-patient. I told them, "You will be in my book!"

I get frustrated very easily because I cannot remember things, feel dizzy lots of the time, and have such a high amount of fatigue. I walk when I can and was even up to five miles a day at one point. I didn't do that much exercise when I was healthy! My taste buds are affected and I still get mouth ulcers, even though I am on an oral chemotherapy routine every other week. I'm still adjusting to taking the chemotherapy for the rest of my life, as Dr. L. told me.

In January 2016, I made an extremely difficult life decision and retired from my job. My last day was January 28. They had a retirement party for me on February 2. I had envisioned being at this job until I retired for real—maybe when I was 70 years old. I absolutely loved what I did as well as the people at ONS. However, the side effects from the chemotherapy drugs, especially fatigue, made it impossible to work full time. I missed the executive work in my part-time role and did not feel like I was doing anything significant. I've always wanted to make a difference for people and make changes for those less fortunate—especially children with special healthcare needs. I did not see those opportunities in this position. Since retiring, I've had several writing opportunities, including finishing this book. I still keep in touch with ONS and am welcome there any time. In fact, they published this book!

I yearn for my regular life, which is now a new life with metastatic cancer. It really sucks, yet it is my only option at this time. Writing this book has helped me see how far I have progressed since those early days. Being a nurse who has become a patient has been one of the hardest things I have ever done. Reliving those years and seeing where I am now is very motivating.

I hope you enjoyed this book and learned a few things along the way. It has been my privilege to share my life with you.

Sincerely,

Elizabeth Wertz Evans

Emevans74@gmail.com

References

Adam, R., Bond, C., & Murchie, P. (2015). Educational interventions for cancer pain. A systematic review of systematic reviews with nested narrative review of randomized controlled trials. *Patient Education and Counseling, 98,* 269–282. doi:10.1016/j.pec.2014.11.003

Aghamohamamdi, A., & Hosseinimehr, S.J. (2016). Natural products for management of oral mucositis induced by radiotherapy and chemotherapy. *Integrative Cancer Therapies, 15,* 60–68. doi:10.1177/1534735415596570

Al-Ansari, S., Zecha, J.A.E., Barasch, A., de Lange, J., Rozema, F.R., & Raber-Durlacher, J.E. (2015). Oral mucositis induced by anticancer therapies. *Current Oral Health Reports, 2,* 202–211. doi:10.1007/s40496-015-0069-4

American Cancer Society. (n.d.). Graphic: New breast cancer screening guideline. Retrieved from http://www.cancer.org/cancer/breastcancer/moreinformation/infographic-new-breast -cancer-screening-guideline

Avery, M., & Williams, F. (2015). The importance of pharmacist providing patient education in oncology. *Journal of Pharmacy Practice, 28,* 26–30. doi:10.1177/0897190014562382

Backman, M., Browall, M., Sundberg, C.J., & Wengström, Y. (2016). Experiencing health—Physical activity during adjuvant chemotherapy treatment for women with breast cancer. *European Journal of Oncology Nursing, 21,* 160–167. doi:10.1016/j.ejon.2015.09.007

Badr, H., Carmack, C.L., Kashy, D.A., Cristofanilli, M., & Revenson, T.A. (2010). Dyadic coping in metastatic breast cancer. *Health Psychology, 29,* 169–180. doi:10.1037/a0018165

Bai, M., Lazenby, M., Jeon, S., Dixon, J., & McCorkle, R. (2015). Exploring the relationship between spiritual well-being and quality of life among patients newly diagnosed with advanced cancer. *Palliative and Supportive Care, 13,* 927–935. doi:10.1017/S1478951514000820

Baker, P., Beesley, H., Fletcher, I., Ablett, J., Holcombe, C., & Salmon, P. (2014). 'Getting back to normal' or 'a new type of normal'? A qualitative study of patients' responses to the existential threat of cancer. *European Journal of Cancer Care, 25,* 180–189. doi:10.1111/ecc.12274

Banning, M. (2011). Employment and breast cancer: A meta-ethnography. *European Journal of Cancer Care, 20,* 708–719. doi:10.1111/j.1365-2354.2011.01291.x

Barnes, A.J., Robert, N., & Bradley, C.J. (2014). Job attributes, job satisfaction and the return to health after breast cancer diagnosis and treatment. *Psycho-Oncology, 23,* 158–164. doi:10.1002/pon.3385

Beach, P.R., & White, B.E. (2013). *In the shadows: How to help your seriously ill adult child.* Pittsburgh, PA: Hygeia Media.

Blanch-Hartigan, D. (2013). Patient satisfaction with physician errors in detecting and identifying patient emotion cues. *Patient Education and Counseling, 93,* 56–62. doi:10.1016/j.pec.2013.04.010

Blaney, J., Lowe-Strong, A., Rankin, J., Campbell, A., Allen, J., & Gracey, J. (2010). The cancer rehabilitation journey: Barriers to and facilitators of exercise among patients with cancer-related fatigue. *Physical Therapy, 90,* 1135–1147. doi:10.2522/ptj.20090278

Brédart, A., Kop, J.-L., Griesser, A.-C., Fiszer, C., Zaman, K., Panes-Ruedin, B., ... Dolbeault, S. (2013). Assessment of needs, health-related quality of life, and satisfaction with care in breast cancer patients to better target supportive care. *Annals of Oncology, 24,* 2151–2158. doi:10.1093/annonc/mdt128

Bride, M.B.M., Neal, L., Dilaveri, C.A., Sandhu, N.P., Hieken, T.J., Ghosh, K., & Wahner-Roedler, D.L. (2013). Factors associated with surgical decision making in women with early-stage breast cancer: A literature review. *Journal of Women's Health, 22,* 236–242. doi:10.1089/jwh.2012.3969

Brocken, P., Prins, J.B., Dekhuijzen, P.N., & van der Heijden, H.F. (2012). The faster the better?—A systematic review on distress in the diagnostic phase of suspected cancer, and the influence of rapid diagnostic pathways. *Psycho-Oncology, 21,* 1–10. doi:10.1002/pon.1929

Brotto, L.A., & Goldmeier, D. (2015). Mindfulness interventions for treating sexual dysfunctions: The gentle science of finding focus in a multitask world. *Journal of Sexual Medicine, 12,* 1687–1689. doi:10.1111/jsm.12941

Brunet, J., Sabiston, C.M., & Burke, S. (2013). Surviving breast cancer: Women's experiences with their changed bodies. *Body Image, 10,* 344–351. doi:10.1016/j.bodyim.2013.02.002

Budden, L.M., Hayes, B.A., & Buettner, P.G. (2014). Women's decision satisfaction and psychological distress following early breast cancer treatment: A treatment decision support role for nurses. *International Journal of Nursing Practice, 20,* 8–16. doi:10.1111/ijn.12243

Butler, L.D., Field, N.P., Busch, A.L., Seplaki, J.E., Hastings, T.A., & Spiegel, D. (2005). Anticipating loss and other temporal stressors predict traumatic stress symptoms among partners of metastatic/recurrent breast cancer patients. *Psycho-Oncology, 14,* 492–502. doi:10.1002/pon.865

Butler, L.D., Koopman, C., Cordova, M.J., Garlan, R.W., DiMiceli, S., & Spiegel, D. (2003). Psychological distress and pain significantly increase before death in metastatic breast cancer patients. *Psychosomatic Medicine, 65,* 416–426. doi:10.1097/01.PSY.0000041472.77692.C6

Canada, A.L., Murphy, P.E., Fitchett, G., & Stein, K. (2016). Re-examining the contributions of faith, meaning, and peace to quality of life: A report from the American Cancer Society's Studies of Cancer Survivors-II (SCS-II). *Annals of Behavioral Medicine, 50,* 79–86. doi:10.1007/s12160-015-9735-y

Caraceni, A., Davies, A., Poulain, P., Cortés-Funes, H., Panchal, S.J., & Fanelli, G. (2013). Guidelines for the management of breakthrough pain in patients with cancer. *Journal of the National Comprehensive Cancer Network, 11*(Suppl. 1), S29–S36. Retrieved from http://www.jnccn.org/content/11/suppl_1/S-29.abstract

Charalampoudis, P., Mantas, D., Sotiropoulos, G.C., Dimitroulis, D., Kouraklis, G., & Markopoulos, C. (2015). Surgery for liver metastases from breast cancer. *Future Oncology, 11,* 1519–1530. doi:10.2217/fon.15.43

Chen, C.H., & Raingruber, B. (2014). Educational needs of inpatient oncology nurses in providing psychosocial care [Online exclusive]. *Clinical Journal of Oncology Nursing, 18,* E1–E5. doi:10.1188/14.CJON.E1-E5

Chlebowski, R.T., Haque, R., Hedlin, H., Col, N., Paskett, E., Manson, J., ... Anderson, G. (2015). Benefit/risk for adjuvant breast cancer therapy with tamoxifen or aromatase inhibitor use by age, and race/ethnicity. *Breast Cancer Research and Treatment, 154,* 609–616. doi:10.1007/s10549-015-3647-1

Choi, E.K., Kim, I.-R., Chang, O., Kang, D., Nam, S.J., Lee, J.E., ... Cho, J. (2014). Impact of chemotherapy-induced alopecia distress on body image, psychosocial well-being, and depression in breast cancer patients. *Psycho-Oncology, 23,* 1103–1110. doi:10.1002/pon.3531

Choo, J., Hutchinson, A., & Bucknall, T. (2010). Nurses' role in medication safety. *Journal of Nursing Management, 18,* 853–861. doi:10.1111/j.1365-2834.2010.01164.x

Chunlestskul, K., Carlson, L.E., Koopmans, J.P., & Angen, M. (2008). Lived experiences of Canadian women with metastatic breast cancer in preparation for their death: A qualitative study. Part I—preparations and consequences. *Journal of Palliative Care, 24,* 5–15.

Coffey, S. (2006). The nurse-patient relationship in cancer care as a shared covenant: A concept analysis. *Advances in Nursing Science, 29,* 308–323. doi:10.1097/00012272-200610000-00005

Collins, A.L., Love, A.W., Bloch, S., Street, A.F., Duchesne, G.M., Dunai, J., & Couper, J.W. (2013). Cognitive existential couple therapy for newly diagnosed prostate cancer patients and their partners: A descriptive pilot study. *Psycho-Oncology, 22,* 465–469. doi:10.1002/pon .2085

Davoll, S., Kowalski, C., Kuhr, K., Ommen, O., Ernstmann, N., & Pfaff, H. (2013). "Tendency to excuse" and patient satisfaction of those suffering with breast cancer. *International Journal of Public Health, 58,* 385–393. doi:10.1007/s00038-012-0405-6

Deschepper, R., Bernheim, J.L., Stichele, R.V., Van den Block, L., Michiels, E., Van Der Kelen, G., ... Deliens, L. (2008). Truth-telling at the end of life: A pilot study on the perspective of patients and professional caregivers. *Patient Education and Counseling, 71,* 52–56. doi:10.1016/j.pec.2007.11.015

Dinc, L., & Gastmans, C. (2013). Trust in nurse-patient relationships: A literature review. *Nursing Ethics, 20,* 501–516. doi:10.1177/0969733012468463

Du, S., Hu, L., Dong, J., Xu, G., Jin, S., Zhang, H., & Yin, H. (2015). Patient education programs for cancer-related fatigue: A systematic review. *Patient Education and Counseling, 98,* 1308–1319. doi:10.1016/j.pec.2015.05.003

Dulisse, B., Li, X., Gayle, J.A., Barron, R.L., Ernst, F.R., Rothman, K.J., ... Kaye, J.A. (2013). A retrospective study of the clinical and economic burden during hospitalizations among cancer patients with febrile neutropenia. *Journal of Medical Economics, 16,* 720–735. doi:10 .3111/13696998.2013.782034

Eichbaum, M.H.R., Kaltwasser, M., Bruckner, T., de Rossi, T.M., Schneeweiss, A., & Sohn, C. (2006). Prognostic factors for patients with liver metastases from breast cancer. *Breast Cancer Research and Treatment, 96,* 53–62. doi:10.1007/s10549-005-9039-1

Fenn, K.M., Evans, S.B., McCorkle, R., DiGiovanna, M.P., Pusztai, L., Sanft, T., ... Chagpar, A.B. (2014). Impact of financial burden of cancer on survivors' quality of life. *Journal of Oncology Practice, 10,* 332–338. doi:10.1200/JOP.2013.001322

Ferraro, C.J., & Catanzaro, P.J. (2011). Radiation therapy. In S.M. Mahon (Ed.), *Site-specific cancer series: Breast cancer* (2nd ed., pp. 105–111). Pittsburgh, PA: Oncology Nursing Society.

Finset, A., Heyn, L., & Ruland, C. (2013). Patterns in clinicians' responses to patient emotion in cancer care. *Patient Education and Counseling, 93,* 80–85. doi:10.1016/j.pec.2013.04.023

Gotink, R.A., Chu, P., Busschbach, J.J., Benson, H., Fricchione, G.L., & Hunink, M.G.M. (2015). Standardised mindfulness-based interventions in healthcare: An overview of systematic reviews and meta-analyses of RCTs. *PLOS ONE, 10,* e0124344. doi:10.1371/journal .pone.0124344

Greenfield, G., Pliskin, J.S., Feder-Bubis, P., Wientroub, S., & Davidovitch, N. (2012). Patient-physician relationships in second opinion encounters—The physicians' perspective. *Social Science and Medicine, 75,* 1202–1212. doi:10.1016/j.socscimed.2012.05.026

Grunfeld, E.A., Low, E., & Cooper, A.F. (2010). Cancer survivors' and employers' perceptions of working following cancer treatment. *Occupational Medicine, 60,* 611–617. doi:10.1093/ occmed/kqq143

Guy, G.P., Jr., Ekwueme, D.U., Yabroff, K.R., Dowling, E.C., Li, C., Rodriguez, J.L., ... Virgo, K.S. (2013). Economic burden of cancer survivorship among adults in the United States. *Journal of Clinical Oncology, 31,* 3749–3757. doi:10.1200/JCO.2013.49.1241

Hack, T.F., & Degner, L.F. (2004). Coping responses following breast cancer diagnosis predict psychological adjustment three years later. *Psycho-Oncology, 13,* 235–247. doi:10.1002/pon.739

Harrison, R., Walton, M., Manias, E., Smith-Merry, J., Kelly, P., Iedema, R., & Robinson, L. (2015). The missing evidence: A systematic review of patients' experiences of adverse events in health care. *International Journal for Quality in Health Care, 27,* 424–442. doi:10.1093/intqhc/mzv075

Hasson-Ohayon, I., Tuval-Mashiach, R., Goldzweig, G., Levi, R., Pizem, N., & Kaufman, B. (2015). The need for friendships and information: Dimensions of social support and posttraumatic growth among women with breast cancer. *Palliative and Supportive Care.* Advance online publication. doi:10.1017/S1478951515001042

Henselmans, I., Fleer, J., de Vries, J., Baas, P.C., Sanderman, R., & Ranchor, A.V. (2010). The adaptive effect of personal control when facing breast cancer: Cognitive and behavioural mediators. *Psychology and Health, 25,* 1023–1040. doi:10.1080/08870440902935921

Husebø, A.M., Allan, H., Karlsen, B., Søreide, J.A., & Bru, E. (2015). Exercise: A path to wellness during adjuvant chemotherapy for breast cancer? *Cancer Nursing, 38,* E13–E20. doi:10.1097/NCC.0000000000000205

Ignatov, A., Hoffman, O., Smith, B., Fahlke, J., Peters, B., Bischoff, J., & Costa, S.-D. (2009). An 11-year retrospective study of totally implanted central venous access ports: Complications and patient satisfaction. *European Journal of Surgical Oncology, 35,* 241–246. doi:10.1016/j.ejso.2008.01.020

Ishida, N., Araki, K., Sakai, T., Kobayashi, K., Kobayashi, T., Fukada, I., ... Yamashita, H. (2015). Fulvestrant 500 mg in postmenopausal patients with metastatic breast cancer: The initial clinical experience. *Breast Cancer.* Advance online publication. doi:10.1007/s12282-015-0612-0

Islam, T., Dahlui, M., Majid, H.A., Nahar, A.M., Mohd Taib, N.A., & Su, T.T. (2014). Factors associated with return to work of breast cancer survivors: A systematic review. *BMC Public Health, 14*(Suppl. 3), S8. doi:10.1186/1471-2458-14-S3-S8

Jafari, N., Zamani, A., Farajzadegan, Z., Bahrami, F., Emami, H., & Loghmani, A. (2013). The effect of spiritual therapy for improving the quality of life of women with breast cancer: A randomized controlled trial. *Psychology, Health, and Medicine, 18,* 56–69. doi:10.1080/13548506.2012.679738

Johnson, K.S., Tulsky, J.A., Hays, J.C., Arnold, R.M., Olsen, M.K., Lindquist, J.H., & Steinhauser, K.E. (2011). Which domains of spirituality are associated with anxiety and depression in patients with advanced illness? *Journal of General Internal Medicine, 26,* 751–758. doi:10.1007/s11606-011-1656-2

Jørgensen, L., Garne, J., Søgaard, M.G., & Laursen, B.S. (2015). The experience of distress in relation to surgical treatment and care for breast cancer: An interview study. *European Journal of Oncology Nursing, 19,* 1–7. doi:101.1016/j.ejon.2015.09.009

Keng, M.K., Thallner, E.A., Elson, P., Ajon, C., Sekeres, J., Wenzell, C.M., ... Sekeres, M.A. (2015). Reducing time to antibiotic administration for febrile neutropenia in the emergency department. *Journal of Oncology Practice, 11,* 450–455. doi:10.1200/JOP.2014.002733

Kent, E.E., Forsythe, L.P., Yabroff, K.R., Weaver, K.E., de Moor, J.S., Rodriguez, J.L., & Rowland, J.H. (2013). Are survivors who report cancer-related financial problems more likely to forgo or delay medical care? *Cancer, 119,* 3710–3717. doi:10.1002/cncr.28262

Kolokotroni, P., Anagnostopoulos, F., & Tsikkinis, A. (2014). Psychosocial factors related to posttraumatic growth in breast cancer survivors: A review. *Women and Health, 54,* 569–592. doi:10.1080/03630242.2014.899543

Kowalski, C., Nitzsche, A., Scheibler, F., Steffen, P., Albert, U.-S., & Pfaff, H. (2009). Breast cancer patients' trust in physicians: The impact of patients' perception of physicians' communication behaviors and hospital organizational climate. *Patient Education and Counseling, 77,* 344–348. doi:10.1016/j.pec.2009.09.003

Kreis, H., Loehberg, C.R., Lux, M.P., Ackermann, S., Lang, W., Beckmann, M.W., & Fasching, P.A. (2007). Patients' attitudes to totally implantable venous access port systems for gynecological or breast malignancies. *European Journal of Surgical Oncology, 33,* 39–43. doi:10.1016/j.ejso.2006.08.003

Krigel, S., Myers, J., Befort, C., Krebill, H., & Klemp, J. (2014). 'Cancer changes everything!' Exploring the lived experiences of women with metastatic breast cancer. *International Journal of Palliative Nursing, 20,* 334–342. doi:10.12968/ijpn.2014.20.7.334

Kroenke, C.H., Quesenberry, C., Kwan, M.L., Sweeney, C., Castillo, A., & Caan, B.J. (2013). Social networks, social support, and burden in relationships, and mortality after breast cancer diagnosis in the Life After Breast Cancer Epidemiology (LACE) study. *Breast Cancer Research and Treatment, 137,* 261–271. doi:10.1007/s10549-012-2253-8

Kutner, J.S., Steiner, J.F., Corbett, K.K., Jahnigen, D.W., & Barton, P.L. (1999). Information needs in terminal illness. *Social Science and Medicine, 48,* 1341–1352. doi:10.1016/S0277-9536(98)00453-5

Lahart, I.M., Metsios, G.S., Nevill, A.M., & Carmichael, A.R. (2015). Physical activity, risk of death and recurrence in breast cancer survivors: A systematic review and meta-analysis of epidemiological studies. *Acta Oncologica, 54,* 635–654. doi:10.3109/0284186X.2014.998275

Lally, R.M. (2010). Acclimating to breast cancer: A process of maintaining self-integrity in the pretreatment period. *Cancer Nursing, 33,* 268–279. doi:10.1097/NCC.0b013e3181d8200b

Lelorain, S., Brédart, A., Dolbeault, S., Cano, A., Bonnaud-Antignac, A., Cousson-Gélie, F., & Sultan, S. (2015). How does a physician's accurate understanding of a cancer patient's unmet needs contribute to patient perception of physician empathy? *Patient Education and Counseling, 98,* 734–741. doi:10.1016/j.pec.2015.03.002

Lepage, C., Smith, A.M., Moreau, J., Barlow-Krelina, E., Wallis, N., Collins, B., … Scherling, C. (2014). A prospective study of grey matter and cognitive function alterations in chemotherapy-treated breast cancer patients. *SpringerPlus, 3,* 444. doi:10.1186/2193-1801-3-444

Leslie, J.L., & Lonneman, W. (2016). Promoting trust in the registered nurse-patient relationship. *Home Healthcare Now, 34,* 38–42. doi:10.1097/nhh.0000000000000322

Leveälahti, H., Tishelman, C., & Öhlén, J. (2007). Framing the onset of lung cancer biographically: Narratives of continuity and disruption. *Psycho-Oncology, 16,* 466–473. doi:10.1002/pon.1080

Lewis, S., Willis, K., Yee, J., & Kilbreath, S. (2016). Living well? Strategies used by women living with metastatic breast cancer. *Qualitative Health Research, 26,* 1167–1179. doi:10.1177/1049732315591787

Lewis, S., Yee, J., Kilbreath, S., & Willis, K. (2015). A qualitative study of women's experiences of healthcare, treatment and support for metastatic breast cancer. *Breast, 24,* 242–247. doi:10.1016/j.breast.2015.02.025

Lyle, B., Landercasper, J., Johnson, J.M., Al-Hamadani, M., Vang, C.A., Groshek, J., … Linebarger, J.H. (2016). Is the American College of Surgeons National Surgical Quality Improvement Program surgical risk calculator applicable for breast cancer patients undergoing breast-conserving surgery? *American Journal of Surgery, 211,* 820–823. doi:10.1016/j.amjsurg.2015.07.013

Manca, G., Rubello, D., Tardelli, E., Giammarile, F., Mazzarri, S., Boni, G., ... Colletti, P.M. (2015). Sentinel lymph node biopsy in breast cancer: Indications, contraindications, and controversies. *Clinical Nuclear Medicine, 41,* 126–133. doi:10.1097/RLU.0000000000000985

Manzi, N.M., Silveira, R.C., & Reis, P.E. (2016). Prophylaxis for mucositis induced by ambulatory chemotherapy: Systematic review. *Journal of Advanced Nursing, 72,* 735–746. doi:10.1111/jan.12867

Mariani, L., Lo Vullo, S., & Bozzetti, F. (2012). Weight loss in cancer patients: A plea for a better awareness of the issue. *Supportive Care in Cancer, 20,* 301–309. doi:10.1007/s00520 -010-1075-7

Martz, C.H., & Kirby, K. (2011). Symptom management. In S.M. Mahon (Ed.), *Site-specific cancer series: Breast cancer* (2nd ed., pp. 141–177). Pittsburgh, PA: Oncology Nursing Society.

Mayer, M. (2010). Lessons learned from the metastatic breast cancer community. *Seminars in Oncology Nursing, 26,* 195–202. doi:10.1016/j.soncn.2010.05.004

McArthur, D., Dumas, A., Woodend, K., Beach, S., & Stacey, D. (2014). Factors influencing adherence to regular exercise in middle-aged women: A qualitative study to inform clinical practice. *BMC Women's Health, 14,* 49. doi:10.1186/1472-6874-14-49

McCabe, C. (2004). Nurse-patient communication: An exploration of patients' experiences. *Journal of Clinical Nursing, 13,* 41–49. doi:10.1111/j.1365-2702.2004.00817.x

McGarvey, E.L., Baum, L.D., Pinkerton, R.C., & Rogers, L.M. (2001). Psychological sequelae and alopecia among women with cancer. *Cancer Practice, 9,* 283–289.

McLaughlin, B., Yoo, W., D'Angelo, J., Tsang, S., Shaw, B., Shah, D., ... Gustafson, D. (2013). It is out of my hands: How deferring control to God can decrease quality of life for breast cancer patients. *Psycho-Oncology, 22,* 2747–2754. doi:10.1002/pon.3356

Mehnert, A., & Koch, U. (2008). Psychological comorbidity and health-related quality of life and its association with awareness, utilization, and need for psychosocial support in a cancer register-based sample of long-term breast cancer survivors. *Journal of Psychosomatic Research, 64,* 383–391. doi:10.1016/j.jpsychores.2007.12.005

Meisel, J.L., Domchek, S.M., Vonderheide, R.H., Giobbie-Hurder, A., Lin, N.U., Winer, E.P., & Partridge, A.H. (2012). Quality of life in long-term survivors of metastatic breast cancer. *Clinical Breast Cancer, 12,* 119–126. doi:10.1016/j.clbc.2012.01.010

Meropol, N.J., Schrag, D., Smith, T.J., Mulvey, T.M., Langdon, R.M., Jr., Blum, D., ... Schnipper, L.E. (2009). American Society of Clinical Oncology guidance statement: The cost of cancer care. *Journal of Clinical Oncology, 27,* 3868–3874. doi:10.1200/ JCO.2009.23.1183

Merrill, A.L., Coopey, S.B., Tang, R., McEvoy, M.P., Specht, M.C., Hughes, K.S., ... Smith, B.L. (2016). Implications of new lumpectomy margin guidelines for breast-conserving surgery: Changes in reexcision rates and predicted rates of residual tumor. *Annals of Surgical Oncology, 23,* 729–736. doi:10.1245/s10434-015-4916-2

Mertz, B.G., Bistrup, P.E., Johansen, C., Dalton, S.O., Deltour, I., Kehlet, H., & Kroman, N. (2012). Psychological distress among women with newly diagnosed breast cancer. *European Journal of Oncology Nursing, 16,* 439–443. doi:10.1016/j.ejon.2011.10.001

Migliorati, C., Hewson, I., Lalla, R., Antunes, H.S., Estilo, C.L., Hodgson, B., ... Elad, S. (2013). Systematic review of laser and other light therapy for the management of oral mucositis in cancer patients. *Supportive Care in Cancer, 21,* 333–341. doi:10.1007/s00520 -012-1605-6

Mikkelsen, T.H., Sondergaard, J., Jensen, A.B., & Olesen, F. (2008). Cancer rehabilitation: Psychosocial rehabilitation needs after discharge from hospital? *Scandinavian Journal of Primary Health Care, 26,* 216–221. doi:10.1080/02813430802295610

Montgomery, M., & McCrone, S.H. (2010). Psychological distress associated with the diagnostic phase for suspected breast cancer: Systematic review. *Journal of Advanced Nursing, 66,* 2372–2390. doi:10.1111/j.1365-2648.2010.05439.x

Moore, C.W., Rauch, P.K., Baer, L., Pirl, W.F., & Muriel, A.C. (2015). Parenting changes in adults with cancer. *Cancer, 121,* 3551–3557. doi:10.1002/cncr.29525

Morgan, S., & Yoder, L.H. (2012). A concept analysis of person-centered care. *Journal of Holistic Nursing, 30,* 6–15. doi:10.1177/0898010111412189

Mosher, C.E., & DuHamel, K.N. (2012). An examination of distress, sleep, and fatigue in metastatic breast cancer patients. *Psycho-Oncology, 21,* 100–107. doi:10.1002/pon.1873

Mosher, C.E., Johnson, C., Dickler, M., Norton, L., Massie, M.J., & DuHamel, K. (2013). Living with metastatic breast cancer: A qualitative analysis of physical, psychological, and social sequelae. *Breast Journal, 19,* 285–292. doi:10.1111/tbj.12107

Moumjid, N., Gafni, A., Bremond, A., & Carrere, M.O. (2007). Seeking a second opinion: Do patients need a second opinion when practice guidelines exist? *Health Policy, 80,* 43–50. doi:10.1016/j.healthpol.2006.02.009

Mustafa, M.K., Bijl, M., & Gans, R. (2002). What is the value of patient-sought second opinions? *European Journal of Internal Medicine, 13,* 445–447. doi:10.1016/S0953-6205(02)00138-3

Nguyen, M.T., Stessin, A., Nagar, H., D'Alfonso, T.M., Chen, Z., Cigler, T., … Shin, S.J. (2014). Impact of Oncotype DX recurrence score in the management of breast cancer cases. *Clinical Breast Cancer, 14,* 182–190. doi:10.1016/j.clbc.2013.12.002

Nilsson, M., Olsson, M., Wennman-Larsen, A., Petersson, L.M., & Alexanderson, K. (2011). Return to work after breast cancer: Women's experiences of encounters with different stakeholders. *European Journal of Oncology Nursing, 15,* 267–274. doi:10.1016/j.ejon.2011.03.005

Niraula, S., Amir, E., Vera-Badillo, F., Seruga, B., Ocana, A., & Tannock, I.F. (2014). Risk of incremental toxicities and associated costs of new anticancer drugs: A meta-analysis. *Journal of Clinical Oncology, 32,* 3634–3642. doi:10.1200/JCO.2014.55.8437

Paiva, C.E., Paiva, B.S.B., de Castro, R.A., de Pádua Souza, C., de Paiva Maia, Y.C., Ayres, J.A., & Michelin, O.C. (2013). A pilot study addressing the impact of religious practice on quality of life of breast cancer patients during chemotherapy. *Journal of Religion and Health, 52,* 184–193. doi:10.1007/s10943-011-9468-6

Park, E.M., Deal, A.M., Check, D.K., Hanson, L.C., Reeder-Hayes, K.E., Mayer, D.K., … Rosenstein, D.L. (2015). Parenting concerns, quality of life, and psychological distress in patients with advanced cancer. *Psycho-Oncology.* Advance online publication. doi:10.1002/pon.3935

Pathak, R., Giri, S., Aryal, M.R., Karmacharya, P., Bhatt, V.R., & Martin, M.G. (2015). Mortality, length of stay, and health care costs of febrile neutropenia-related hospitalizations among patients with breast cancer in the United States. *Supportive Care in Cancer, 23,* 615–617. doi:10.1007/s00520-014-2553-0

Paulson, S., Davidson, R., Jha, A., & Kabat-Zinn, J. (2013). Becoming conscious: The science of mindfulness. *Annals of the New York Academy of Sciences, 1303,* 87–104. doi:10.1111/nyas.12203

Payne, V.L., Singh, H., Meyer, A.N., Levy, L., Harrison, D., & Graber, M.L. (2014). Patient-initiated second opinions: Systematic review of characteristics and impact on diagnosis, treatment, and satisfaction. *Mayo Clinic Proceedings, 89,* 687–696. doi:10.1016/j.mayocp.2014.02.015

Porensky, E.K., & Carpenter, B.D. (2015). Breaking bad news: Effects of forecasting diagnosis and framing prognosis. *Patient Education and Counseling, 99,* 68–76. doi:10.1016/j.pec.2015.07.022

Raupach, J.C., & Hiller, J.E. (2002). Information and support for women following the primary treatment of breast cancer. *Health Expectations, 5,* 289–301. doi:10.1046/j.1369-6513.2002.00191.x

Reinbolt, R.E., Mangini, N., Hill, J.L., Levine, L.B., Dempsey, J.L., Singaravelu, J., … Lustberg, M.B. (2015). Endocrine therapy in breast cancer: The neoadjuvant, adjuvant, and metastatic approach. *Seminars in Oncology Nursing, 31,* 146–155. doi:10.1016/j.soncn.2015.02.002

Reinert, T., & Barrios, C.H. (2015). Optimal management of hormone receptor positive metastatic breast cancer in 2016. *Therapeutic Advances in Medical Oncology, 7,* 304–320. doi:10.1177/1758834015608993

Rhondali, W., Chisholm, G.B., Daneshmand, M., Allo, J., Kang, D.-H., Filbet, M., … Bruera, E. (2013). Association between body image dissatisfaction and weight loss among patients with advanced cancer and their caregivers: A preliminary report. *Journal of Pain and Symptom Management, 45,* 1039–1049. doi:10.1016/j.jpainsymman.2012.06.013

Richardson, A. (2004). Creating a culture of compassion: Developing supportive care for people with cancer. *European Journal of Oncology Nursing, 8,* 293–305. doi:10.1016/j.ejon.2004.07.004

Roe, H. (2011). Chemotherapy-induced alopecia: Advice and support for hair loss. *British Journal of Nursing, 20,* S4–S12. doi:10.12968/bjon.2011.20.Sup5.S4

Rose, S.L., Spencer, R.J., & Rausch, M.M. (2013). The use of humor in patients with recurrent ovarian cancer: A phenomenological study. *International Journal of Gynecological Cancer, 23,* 775–779. doi:10.1097/IGC.0b013e31828addd5

Runowicz, C.D., Leach, C.R., Henry, N.L., Henry, K.S., Mackey, H.T., Cowens-Alvarado, R.L., … Ganz, P.A. (2016). American Cancer Society/American Society of Clinical Oncology breast cancer survivorship care guideline. *Journal of Clinical Oncology, 34,* 611–635. doi:10.1200/JCO.2015.64.3809

Ruthig, J.C., & Holfeld, B. (2016). Positive thinking and social perceptions of a male vs. female peer's cancer experience. *Journal of Social Psychology, 156,* 154–167. doi:10.1080/00224545.2015.1052361

Ruthig, J.C., Holfeld, B., & Hanson, B.L. (2012). The role of positive thinking in social perceptions of cancer outcomes. *Psychology and Health, 27,* 1244–1258. doi:10.1080/08870446.2012.666549

Saif, M.W., Katirtzoglou, N.A., & Syrigos, K.N. (2008). Capecitabine: An overview of the side effects and their management. *Anticancer Drugs, 19,* 447–464.

Sandberg, J.C., Strom, C., & Arcury, T.A. (2014). Strategies used by breast cancer survivors to address work-related limitations during and after treatment. *Women's Health Issues, 24,* e197–e204. doi:10.1016/j.whi.2013.12.007

Sarenmalm, E.K., Thorén-Jönsson, A.L., Gaston-Johansson, F., & Öhlén, J. (2009). Making sense of living under the shadow of death: Adjusting to a recurrent breast cancer illness. *Qualitative Health Research, 19,* 1116–1130. doi:10.1177/1049732309341728

Schirrmacher, V., Stücker, W., Lulei, M., Bihari, A.S., & Sprenger, T. (2015). Long-term survival of a breast cancer patient with extensive liver metastases upon immune and virotherapy: A case report. *Immunotherapy, 7,* 855–860. doi:10.2217/imt.15.48

Schmid-Büchi, S., van den Borne, B., Dassen, T., & Halfens, R.J.G. (2011). Factors associated with psychosocial needs of close relatives of women under treatment for breast cancer. *Journal of Clinical Nursing, 20,* 1115–1124. doi:10.1111/j.1365-2702.2010.03376.x

Schreiber, J.A. (2011). Image of God: Effect on coping and psychospiritual outcomes in early breast cancer survivors. *Oncology Nursing Forum, 38,* 293–301. doi:10.1188/11.ONF.293 -301

Schreiber, J.A., & Edward, J. (2015). Image of God, religion, spirituality, and life changes in breast cancer survivors: A qualitative approach. *Journal of Religion and Health, 54,* 612–622. doi:10.1007/s10943-014-9862-y

Segrin, C., & Badger, T.A. (2014). Psychological and physical distress are interdependent in breast cancer survivors and their partners. *Psychology Health and Medicine, 19,* 716–723. doi: 10.1080/13548506.2013.871304

Seidensticker, M., Garlipp, B., Scholz, S., Mohnike, K., Popp, F., Steffen, I., ... Ricke, J. (2015). Locally ablative treatment of breast cancer liver metastases: Identification of factors influencing survival (the Mammary Cancer Microtherapy and Interventional Approaches [MAMMA MIA] study). *BMC Cancer, 15,* 517. doi:10.1186/s12885-015-1499-z

Shapiro, J.P., McCue, K., Heyman, E.N., Dey, T., & Haller, H.S. (2010). Coping-related variables associated with individual differences in adjustment to cancer. *Journal of Psychosocial Oncology, 28,* 1–22. doi:10.1080/07347330903438883

Shigematsu, N., Takeda, A., Sanuki, N., Fukada, J., Uno, T., Ito, H., ... Kubo, A. (2006). Radiation therapy after breast-conserving surgery. *Radiation Medicine, 24,* 388–404. doi:10.1007/ s11604-005-0021-y

Shin, H., Jo, S.J., Kim do, H., Kwon, O., & Myung, S.K. (2015). Efficacy of interventions for prevention of chemotherapy-induced alopecia: A systematic review and meta-analysis. *International Journal of Cancer, 136,* E442–E454. doi:10.1002/ijc.29115

Smeulers, M., Onderwater, A.T., van Zwieten, M.C., & Vermeulen, H. (2014). Nurses' experiences and perspectives on medication safety practices: An explorative qualitative study. *Journal of Nursing Management, 22,* 276–285. doi:10.1111/jonm.12225

Soo, H., & Sherman, K.A. (2015). Rumination, psychological distress and post-traumatic growth in women diagnosed with breast cancer. *Psycho-Oncology, 24,* 70–79. doi:10.1002/ pon.3596

Sousa, A.M., de Santana Neto, J., Guimaraes, G.M., Cascudo, G.M., Neto, J.O., & Ashmawi, H.A. (2014). Safety profile of intravenous patient-controlled analgesia for breakthrough pain in cancer patients: A case series study. *Supportive Care in Cancer, 22,* 795–801. doi:10.1007/s00520-013-2036-8

Sprung, B.R., Janotha, B.L., & Steckel, A.J. (2011). The lived experience of breast cancer patients and couple distress. *Journal of the American Academy of Nurse Practitioners, 23,* 619–627. doi:10.1111/j.1745-7599.2011.00653.x

Swarm, R.A., Abernethy, A.P., Anghelescu, D.L., Benedetti, C., Buga, S., Cleeland, C., ... Kumar, R. (2013). Adult cancer pain. *Journal of the National Comprehensive Cancer Network, 11,* 992–1022. Retrieved from http://www.jnccn.org/content/11/8/992.abstract

Tanay, M.A., Roberts, J., & Ream, E. (2013). Humour in adult cancer care: A concept analysis. *Journal of Advanced Nursing, 69,* 2131–2140. doi:10.1111/jan.12059

Tanco, K., Rhondali, W., Perez-Cruz, P., Tanzi, S., Chisholm, G.B., Baile, W., ... Bruera, E. (2015). Patient perception of physician compassion after a more optimistic vs. a less optimistic message: A randomized clinical trial. *JAMA Oncology, 1,* 176–183. doi:10.1001/jam aoncol.2014.297

Taniyama, T.K., Hashimoto, K., Katsumata, N., Hirakawa, A., Yonemori, K., Yunokawa, M., ... Fujiwara, Y. (2014). Can oncologists predict survival for patients with progressive disease after standard chemotherapies? *Current Oncology, 21,* 84–90. doi:10.3747/ co.21.1743

Tasmuth, T., von Smitten, K., & Kalso, E. (1996). Pain and other symptoms during the first year after radical and conservative surgery for breast cancer. *British Journal of Cancer, 74,* 2024–2031. doi:10.1038/bjc.1996.671

Tate, D.F., Lyons, E.J., & Valle, C.G. (2015). High-tech tools for exercise motivation: Use and role of technologies such as the internet, mobile applications, social media, and video games. *Diabetes Spectrum, 28,* 45–54. doi:10.2337/diaspect.28.1.45

Tattersall, M.H., Dear, R.F., Jansen, J., Shepherd, H.L., Devine, R.J., Horvath, L.G., & Boyer, M.L. (2009). Second opinions in oncology: The experiences of patients attending the Sydney Cancer Centre. *Medical Journal of Australia, 191,* 209–212.

Thorne, S.E., Oliffe, J.L., Oglov, V., & Gelmon, K. (2013). Communication challenges for chronic metastatic cancer in an era of novel therapeutics. *Qualitative Health Research, 23,* 863–875. doi:10.1177/1049732313483926

Tiedtke, C., de Rijk, A., Donceel, P., Christiaens, M.R., & de Casterlé, B.D. (2012). Survived but feeling vulnerable and insecure: A qualitative study of the mental preparation for RTW after breast cancer treatment. *BMC Public Health, 12,* 538. doi:10.1186/1471-2458-12-538

Tirodkar, M.A., Acciavatti, N., Roth, L.M., Stovall, E., Nasso, S.F., Sprandio, J., … Scholle, S.H. (2015). Lessons from early implementation of a patient-centered care model in oncology. *Journal of Oncology Practice, 11,* 456–461. doi:10.1200/JOP.2015.006072

Trinh, L., Mutrie, N., Campbell, A.M., Crawford, J.J., & Courneya, K.S. (2014). Effects of supervised exercise on motivational outcomes in breast cancer survivors at 5-year follow-up. *European Journal of Oncology Nursing, 18,* 557–563. doi:10.1016/j.ejon.2014.07.004

Umezawa, S., Fujimori, M., Matsushima, E., Kinoshita, H., & Uchitomi, Y. (2015). Preferences of advanced cancer patients for communication on anticancer treatment cessation and the transition to palliative care. *Cancer, 121,* 4240–4249. doi:10.1002/cncr.29635

U.S. Preventive Services Task Force. (2016). Breast cancer: Screening. Retrieved from http://www.uspreventiveservicestaskforce.org/Page/Document/UpdateSummaryFinal/breast-cancer-screening1?ds=1&s=screening%20breast%20cancer

Valenti, R.B. (2014). Chemotherapy education for patients with cancer: A literature review. *Clinical Journal of Oncology Nursing, 18,* 637–640. doi:10.1188/14.CJON.637-640

Van Sebille, Y.Z.A., Stansborough, R., Wardill, H.R., Bateman, E., Gibson, R.J., & Keefe, D.M. (2015). Management of mucositis during chemotherapy: From pathophysiology to pragmatic therapeutics. *Current Oncology Reports, 17,* 50. doi:10.1007/s11912-015-0474-9

Veselka, L., Schermer, J.A., Martin, R.A., & Vernon, P.A. (2010). Laughter and resiliency: A behavioral genetic study of humor styles and mental toughness. *Twin Research and Human Genetics, 13,* 442–449. doi:10.1375/twin.13.5.442

Vidall, C., Fernández-Ortega, P., Cortinovis, D., Jahn, P., Amlani, B., & Scotté, F. (2015). Impact and management of chemotherapy/radiotherapy-induced nausea and vomiting and the perceptual gap between oncologists/oncology nurses and patients: A cross-sectional multinational survey. *Supportive Care in Cancer, 23,* 3297–3305. doi:10.1007/s00520-015-2750-5

Vilhauer, R.P. (2008). A qualitative study of the experiences of women with metastatic breast cancer. *Palliative and Supportive Care, 6,* 249–258. doi:10.1017/S1478951508000382

Virizuela, J.A., Carratalà, J., Aguado, J.M., Vicente, D., Salavert, M., Ruiz, M., … Cruz, J.J. (2016). Management of infection and febrile neutropenia in patients with solid cancer. *Clinical and Translational Oncology, 18,* 557–570. doi:10.1007/s12094-015-1442-4

Von Ah, D., Habermann, B., Carpenter, J.S., & Schneider, B.L. (2013). Impact of perceived cognitive impairment in breast cancer survivors. *European Journal of Oncology Nursing, 17,* 236–241. doi:10.1016/j.ejon.2012.06.002

Wälivaara, B.M., Sävenstedt, S., & Axelsson, K. (2013). Caring relationships in home-based nursing care—Registered nurses' experiences. *Open Nursing Journal, 7,* 89–95.

Waller, A., Forshaw, K., Bryant, J., Carey, M., Boyes, A., & Sanson-Fisher, R. (2015). Preparatory education for cancer patients undergoing surgery: A systematic review of volume and quality of research output over time. *Patient Education and Counseling, 98,* 1540–1549. doi:10.1016/j.pec.2015.05.008

Warren, M. (2009). Metastatic breast cancer recurrence: A literature review of themes and issues arising from diagnosis. *International Journal of Palliative Nursing, 15,* 222–225. Retrieved from http://search.ebscohost.com/login.aspx?direct=true&db=c8h&AN=2010313195&site=ehost-live

Warren, M. (2010). Uncertainty, lack of control and emotional functioning in women with metastatic breast cancer: A review and secondary analysis of the literature using the critical appraisal technique. *European Journal of Cancer Care, 19,* 564–574. doi:10.1111/j.1365-2354.2010.01215.x

Watson, M., Homewood, J., & Haviland, J. (2012). Coping response and survival in breast cancer patients: A new analysis. *Stress and Health, 28,* 376–380. doi:10.1002/smi.2459

Watts, R., Botti, M., & Hunter, M. (2010). Nurses' perspectives on the care provided to cancer patients. *Cancer Nursing, 33,* E1–E8. doi:10.1097/NCC.0b013e3181b5575a

Weiss, T. (2004). Correlates of posttraumatic growth in married breast cancer survivors. *Journal of Social and Clinical Psychology, 23,* 733–746. doi:10.1521/jscp.23.5.733.50750

Wiechula, R., Conroy, T., Kitson, A.L., Marshall, R.J., Whitaker, N., & Rasmussen, P. (2016). Umbrella review of the evidence: What factors influence the caring relationship between a nurse and patient? *Journal of Advanced Nursing, 72,* 723–734. doi:10.1111/jan.12862

Wilkinson, S., & Kitzinger, C. (2000). Thinking differently about thinking positive: A discursive approach to cancer patients' talk. *Social Science and Medicine, 50,* 797–811. doi:10.1016/S0277-9536(99)00337-8

Wittenberg-Lyles, E., Goldsmith, J., & Ferrell, B. (2013). Oncology nurse communication barriers to patient-centered care. *Clinical Journal of Oncology Nursing, 17,* 152–158. doi:10.1188/13.CJON.152-158

Würtzen, H., Dalton, S.O., Christensen, J., Andersen, K.K., Elsass, P., Flyger, H.L., … Johansen, C. (2015). Effect of mindfulness-based stress reduction on somatic symptoms, distress, mindfulness and spiritual wellbeing in women with breast cancer: Results of a randomized controlled trial. *Acta Oncologica, 54,* 712–719. doi:10.3109/0284186X.2014.997371

Xiao, W., Chow, K.M., So, W.K.W., Leung, D.Y., & Chan, C.W.H. (2015). The effectiveness of psychoeducational intervention on managing symptom clusters in patients with cancer: A systematic review of randomized controlled trials. *Cancer Nursing.* Advance online publication. doi:10.1097/NCC.0000000000000313

Yabroff, K.R., Dowling, E.C., Guy, G.P., Jr., Banegas, M.P., Davidoff, A., Han, X., … Ekwueme, D.U. (2015). Financial hardship associated with cancer in the United States: Findings from a population-based sample of adult cancer survivors. *Journal of Clinical Oncology, 34,* 259–267. doi:10.1200/JCO.2015.62.0468

Yackzan, S. (2011). Pathophysiology and staging. In S.M. Mahon (Ed.), *Site-specific cancer series: Breast cancer* (2nd ed., pp. 65–77). Pittsburgh, PA: Oncology Nursing Society.

Yackzan, S., & Hatch, J. (2011). Surgical management and reconstruction. In S.M. Mahon (Ed.), *Site-specific cancer series: Breast cancer* (2nd ed., pp. 79–103). Pittsburgh, PA: Oncology Nursing Society.

Yu, L.S., Chojniak, R., Borba, M.A., Girão, D.S., & Lourenço, M.T. (2011). Prevalence of anxiety in patients awaiting diagnostic procedures in an oncology center in Brazil. *Psycho-Oncology, 20,* 1242–1245. doi:10.1002/pon.1842

Ziner, K.W., Sledge, G.W., Bell, C.J., Johns, S., Miller, K.D., & Champion, V.L. (2012). Predicting fear of breast cancer recurrence and self-efficacy in survivors by age at diagnosis. *Oncology Nursing Forum, 39,* 287–295. doi:10.1188/12.ONF.287-295

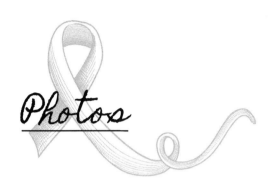

Photos

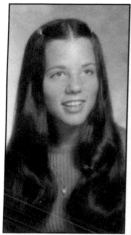

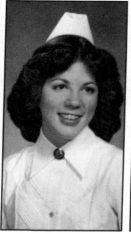

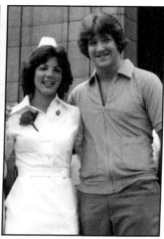

June 1974—My senior picture from high school

1980—My graduation from the St. Francis General Hospital School of Nursing

1980—Pat and me at my nursing graduation

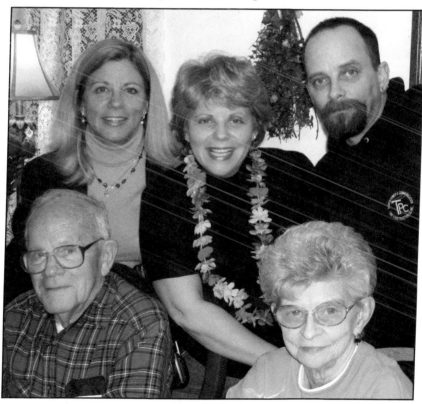

My nuclear family
(From left to right) Front row: My dad Bill and my mom Helen. Back row: Me, my sister Patty, and my brother Charlie

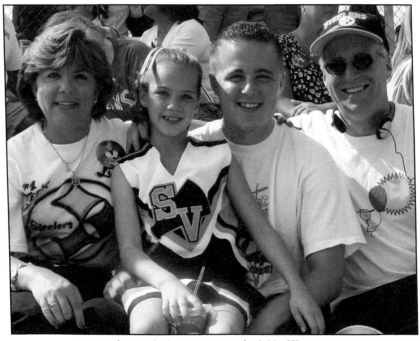

An outside cheer competition for Ashley Wertz
From left to right: Me, Ashley Wertz, Patrick, and Pat

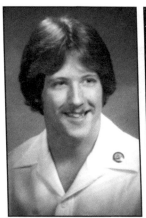

1981—Pat's graduation from nursing school

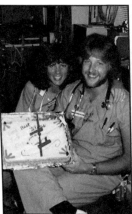

1983—Throwing a going-away party for Pat when he left the cardiovascular intensive care unit to become a flight nurse. I made the cake and put a toy helicopter on it!

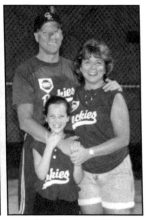

2002—Pat was Ashley's coach for softball. I was the scorekeeper.

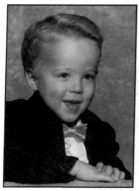

A young Patrick serving as
ring bearer at a wedding for
family friends

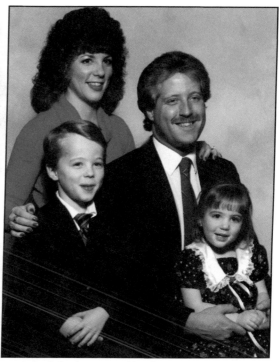

1989—A family portrait of Pat, Patrick, Amanda, and me
around Christmas time

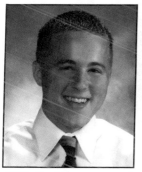

2002—Patrick's senior year of
high school

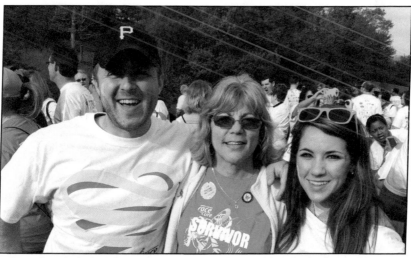

2014—Patrick, Ashley Wertz, and me at the Susan G. Komen Race for the Cure on Mother's
Day. I was diagnosed with metastatic cancer to my liver about two weeks later.

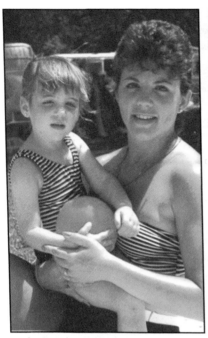

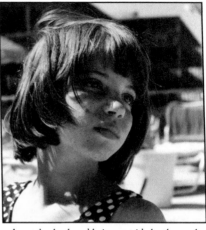

Amanda also loved being outside by the pool.

A young Amanda and me on one of our camping trips. Our swimsuits kind of matched!

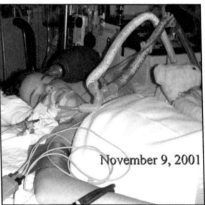

November 9, 2001

Amanda was only 14 years old when she died from multiple medical errors in the hospital.

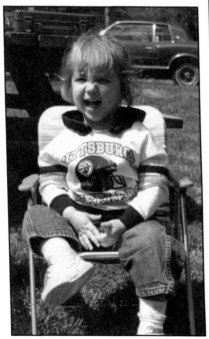

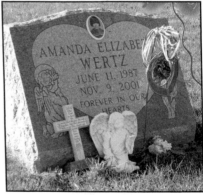

Amanda loved camping when she was little.

We miss Amanda so much!

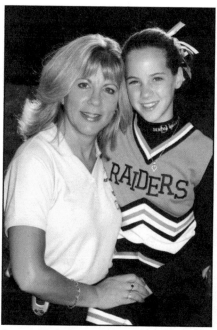

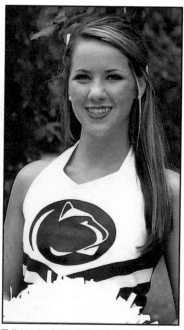

I was Ashley's cheerleading coach for her teams in 2004 through 2005. All she wanted after the crash was for her legs to heal so she could cheer again.

Fall 2015—Ashley Wertz, Penn State senior and cheerleader

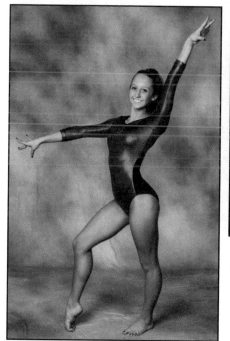

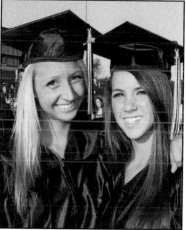

Above
2011—Ashley Evans' (left) and Ashley Wertz's (right) graduation from high school

---

Left
Ashley Evans was a gymnast from age 7 through high school.

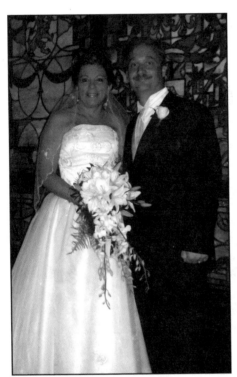

Left
September 8, 2007—Hipp and me on
our wedding day

July 11, 2009—Standing with Dayna,
who received Amanda's liver in 2001.
After Amanda's death, we donated as
many of her organs as we could.

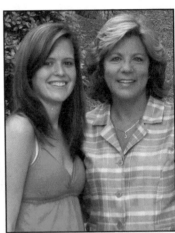

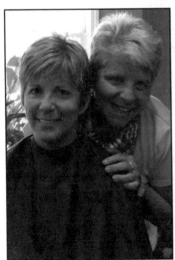

Smiling with Patty after getting my hair
cut short. It made the process of losing it
all during chemotherapy a bit easier.

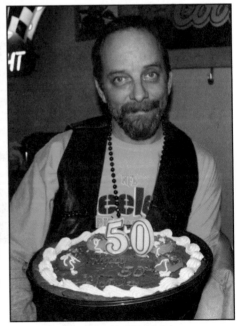

Charlie on his 50th birthday

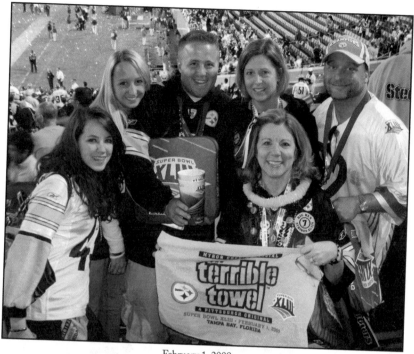

February 1, 2009—
The family at Super Bowl XLIII in Tampa, Florida. This picture was after the Steelers won Super Bowl 43!
(From left to right) Front row: Ashley Wertz and me. Back row: Ashley Evans, Patrick, my sister-in-law Sharon Wood, and Hipp

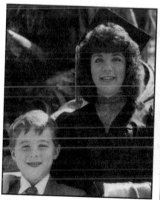

May 1996—Patrick and me at my graduation from Carnegie Mellon University. I received a master's of public management degree.

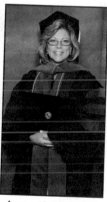

August 13, 2013—My graduation from Capella University for my PhD!

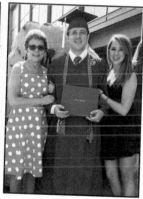

May 15, 2015—Celebrating Patrick's graduation from Duquesne University with Ashley Wertz

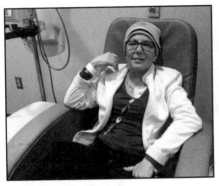

Receiving a chemotherapy treatment

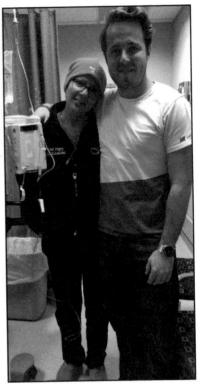

Patrick and me during a chemotherapy infusion

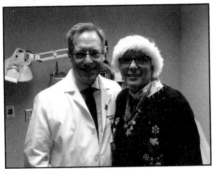

Dr. L. is my oncologist through the Hillman Cancer Center in Pittsburgh. He is VERY patient-oriented and has explained the good and the bad of metastasis.

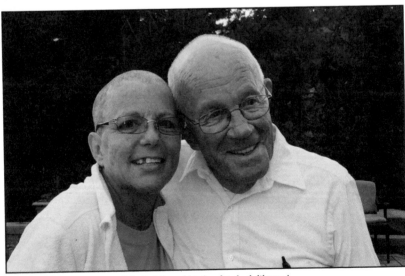

My dad shaved his head to look like me!